Musculoskeletal Practice:
A quick reference guide for allied health professionals in primary care

Primary Care Essentials

Series Editor: Georgette Eaton

The Primary Care Essentials series brings together a selection of subject-specific books which reflect the curriculum for work in primary care. These books are written specifically for the wide range of clinicians and associated professionals involved in the primary care setting and offer accessible, visual and evidence-based guidance on specific topics you may come across as part of your role.

Bringing together a multi-professional team of authors, these quick-reference resources are specifically written to support non-specialists and are ideal for double checking your knowledge whenever you need to. Whether you are a nurse, physician associate, midwife, paramedic, physiotherapist, pharmacist, or social prescriber, it provides all the essential information you need in one place, so you can feel more confident navigating your way around the breadth and complexities of the primary care role.

Musculoskeletal Practice:
A quick reference guide for allied health professionals in primary care

Sampada Bhide

CLASS PROFESSIONAL

Printing history
This first edition published in 2026.

The authors and publisher welcome feedback from the users of this book.
Please contact the publisher:

Class Professional,
The Exchange, Express Park, Bristol Road, Bridgwater TA6 4RR

Telephone: 01278 472 800
Email: info@class.co.uk
Website: www.classprofessional.co.uk

Class Professional is an imprint of Class Publishing Ltd
A CIP catalogue record for this book is available from the British Library

Paperback ISBN: 9781801611282
ePub: 9781801611305
ePDF: 9781801611299

Cover design by Nicky Borowiec.

Designed and typeset by PHi Business Solutions
Printed in the UK by Hobbs

This book is printed on paper from responsible sources. Refer to local recycling guidance on disposal of this book.

Product safety information can be found at https://www.classprofessional.co.uk/terms-of-use/gpsr-statement/

MIX
Paper | Supporting responsible forestry
FSC® C020438
www.fsc.org

CARBON BALANCED PRINT
www.carbonbalancedprint.com
CBP2250

Contents

List of Figures

List of Tables

About the Authors

Sampada 'Sam' Bhide is an Advanced Physiotherapy Practitioner with over 18 years of clinical experience in musculoskeletal (MSK) medicine, primary care and rheumatology. She holds a Master's degree in Musculoskeletal Physiotherapy and is an Independent Prescriber, enabling her to assess, diagnose, request investigations, prescribe medication and deliver comprehensive management for complex MSK presentations.

Sam has worked at an advanced clinical level within primary care, managing complex spinal conditions, inflammatory rheumatological disorders, persistent pain and multi-factorial musculoskeletal presentations. Her practice integrates evidence-based medicine with a strong biopsychosocial framework, emphasising personalised care, shared decision-making and patient empowerment.

She is the Founder and Clinical Director of Physiozen Ltd., a holistic physiotherapy and wellness clinic in Surrey, where she leads a multidisciplinary approach combining physiotherapy, Pilates, movement rehabilitation and digital innovation to improve long-term patient outcomes.

Alongside clinical practice, Sam is actively involved in professional leadership and education. She serves on executive committees within national MSK organisations, contributes to consensus and guideline development in rheumatology and is a peer reviewer for academic journals. She is a conference speaker, educator, and mentor and guest lecturer on first-contact physiotherapy courses supporting the development of advanced practice physiotherapists across the UK.

Sam's work has been recognised with multiple professional awards for innovation, leadership and contribution to physiotherapy practice. Her clinical interests include complex spine care, rheumatology, persistent pain, hormonal influences in MSK health and advancing the role of physiotherapists within primary care medicine.

This book reflects her commitment to strengthening clinical reasoning, raising standards in MSK assessment and supporting clinicians to practise with confidence, clarity and compassion.

Christopher 'Chris' Martey is a Chartered Physiotherapist, injection therapist and non-medical prescriber working as a Musculoskeletal (MSK) Transformation Clinical Lead in Primary Care and Urgent Primary Care. Chris complements his clinical role with a leadership position as a Multi-Professional Primary and Community Care Education Lead. With a passion for Rheumatic and MSK Diseases (RMDs) since working as a Senior Physiotherapist in Rheumatology at the Royal National Hospital for Rheumatic Diseases, Chris maintains his specialism as a member of the European Alliance of Associations for Rheumatology (EULAR) Health Professionals in Rheumatology (HPR) Committee and education subcommittee. Chris is also a Primary Care MSK Core Skills Trainer with Arthritis UK and has a keen interest in healthcare leadership, strategy and policy. He is also the Chair of the Board of Trustees for the Arthritis and Musculoskeletal Alliance (ARMA).

A Note from the Author

The development of *Musculoskeletal Practice: A quick reference guide for allied health professionals in primary care* is rooted in the dynamic changes taking place within primary care, particularly as reflected in the NHS Improvement Plan. My dedication as a physiotherapist has always centred on a strong enthusiasm for the musculoskeletal system. The remarkable complexity of the human body continues to inspire my professional curiosity, driving a lifelong commitment to better understand its intricacies.

Throughout my career, I have been guided by the conviction that the optimal way to address the challenges presented by musculoskeletal conditions is through attentive listening to patients, empowering them to understand their bodies and supporting their journey towards optimal function. My guiding principle is simple yet profound: to treat every patient in the manner I would wish to be treated myself – with unwavering compassion and respect. This philosophy has informed my practice across both NHS and private healthcare settings.

Over time, it became evident that healthcare professionals in primary care required a resource that is both concise and comprehensive to support the diagnosis and management of musculoskeletal conditions. This book has been created specifically to meet that need. It provides a structured and practical framework designed to adopt clinical reasoning, pattern recognition and effective management strategies for musculoskeletal conditions encountered in primary care environments. My hope is that this guide will serve as a valuable companion throughout your professional career.

Acknowledgements

I wish to extend my heartfelt thanks to Chris Martey for his considerable contribution to the rheumatology chapter. I am also deeply grateful to my family, whose unwavering support has made it possible for me to embark on and complete this project. Lastly, I would like to acknowledge the encouragement and assistance provided by Class Professional for bringing this vision to fruition.

Introduction

Scope and Purpose

Musculoskeletal (MSK) health conditions represent a significant proportion of presentations in primary care, with approximately one in six GP consultations seeking advice and management for issues affecting the joints, bones, soft tissues, muscles and nerves (Hill et al., 2022). MSK disorders affect individuals physically, mentally, socially and financially (Blyth et al., 2019; Versus Arthritis, 2023). This guide has been developed specifically for primary care professionals, including general practitioners (GPs), nurses, allied healthcare professionals (AHPs), first-contact practitioners (FCPs) and advanced practitioners (APs).

Aims

The principal objective of this book is to support clinicians in the identification, assessment, safety netting, management and appropriate referral of patients experiencing MSK conditions. It is grounded in evidence-based literature and offers a comprehensive overview of the most common MSK presentations encountered within clinical practice.

Focus and Content Selection

Rather than attempting to cover the full spectrum of MSK diagnoses, this guide concentrates on the conditions most frequently seen in primary care. The conditions are selected based on their prevalence and relevance and the challenges they present in diagnosis, ensuring that the information provided is practical and applicable for daily clinical use. While the guide offers a structured approach to diagnosis, assessment and management, it is not exhaustive. For rare or particularly complex cases, readers are advised to consult specialist resources or advanced MSK textbooks for further detail.

Practical Application

Through the provision of a structured and practical framework, this guide aims to enhance clinical reasoning, pattern recognition, safety netting and decision-making processes related to MSK conditions. Whether utilised as a reference for daily practice or as a resource for further study, this guide is designed to simplify clinical decision making and promote the effective delivery of MSK healthcare.

CHAPTER 1

Structured Approach to Musculoskeletal Consultations

Musculoskeletal (MSK) consultations require a logical and systematic structure to ensure effective patient care. The consultation process encompasses the collection of both subjective and objective information, with a strong emphasis on integrating the patient's own perspective throughout. By doing so, clinicians can formulate a well-founded clinical hypothesis that guides subsequent assessment and management. This approach aligns with recommendations from the National Institute for Health and Care Excellence (NICE, 2022a) and provides a foundation for high-quality clinical decision making.

The key elements of a structured MSK consultation, as outlined by the Academy of Physical Medicine (2018), are as follows.

- **Gathering subjective information:** Elicit the patient's history, including history of presenting complaint, onset, duration, progression of symptoms, as well as relevant medical, social and occupational factors.
- **Collecting objective data:** Perform a focused physical examination to obtain clinical findings that support or refute possible diagnoses.
- **Integrating patient perspectives:** Consider the patient's views, concerns and expectations regarding their condition and treatment preferences.
- **Formulating a clinical hypothesis:** Process the gathered information to develop a working diagnosis, which will inform the next steps in management and, if appropriate, guide further investigations or referral.

Adhering to this structured approach ensures that MSK consultations are comprehensive, patient centred and conducive to accurate diagnosis and effective management.

Shared Decision Making in Musculoskeletal Consultations

The NICE guideline NG197 (NICE, 2021a) defines shared decision making as a process in which healthcare professionals and patients work together to make informed care decisions based on beliefs, preferences and priorities.

Musculoskeletal conditions often require patients to actively manage fluctuating symptoms. Shared decision making is essential in MSK practice, as it helps patients understand their diagnosis, condition progression and treatment options like exercise, medications, activity changes, injections and onward referrals. Musculoskeletal care seldom involves a universally optimal intervention, so incorporating patient preferences and objectives is essential for effective management. Involving patients through shared decision making improves adherence to treatment and confidence in self-management and reduces unnecessary referrals.

This approach supports the principle of 'No decision about me without me' by empowering and involving patients. According to NICE NG197, integrating shared decision making enhances communication, outcomes and person-centred MSK care (NICE, 2021a).

Key Considerations in Musculoskeletal Assessments

A thorough understanding of the characteristics of pain is essential in MSK assessments, as the nature of the pain can significantly influence the diagnostic process. The following outlines the most common pain patterns encountered in MSK clinical practice, offering guidance for effective clinical reasoning and decision making (Bennett et al., 2016; Salisbury et al., 2022a).

Pain Characteristics and Patterns

- **Ache, throbbing or dull pain:** These sensations are frequently associated with muscular and tendinous structures. Such pain often worsens with loading and overuse. For instance, tennis elbow is a classic example in which repetitive strain on the tendons leads to a persistent, aching discomfort (Dijkstra et al., 2020).
- **Sharp pain, electric shock-like sensations, pins and needles, tingling, numbness or stabbing pain:** These symptoms are suggestive of nerve involvement. Typically, this type of pain intensifies with compression or movement of the affected body part, as seen in conditions such as sciatica (lumbar radiculopathy). The presence of these descriptors should prompt consideration of neuropathic pain pathways (Zusman et al., 2022).
- **Deep bone pain:** Pain that feels deep is most noticeable during loading/weight-bearing activities. For example, in cases of osteoarthritis affecting the hip or knee joints, patients often report discomfort when walking or running, indicating involvement of the underlying bony structures (McCormick et al., 2020).
- **Constant pain (not relieved by positional change):** Persistent pain that does not respond to changes in position may be indicative of visceral

pathology or other serious underlying conditions. Such clinical presentations necessitate prompt escalation and further diagnostic evaluation to exclude potential serious diagnoses (Turnpenney et al., 2015).

Conducting an Effective Musculoskeletal Assessment

Introduce Yourself and Your Role and Confirm Patient Details

This is essential for medicolegal purposes and building good rapport with the patient (Freeman et al., 2002).

Elicit the Chief Complaint

Encourage detailed symptom description by asking 'How can I help?'.

It is important to encourage the patient to describe their symptoms in detail, allowing them to speak without interruption. This approach provides patients with the space to fully express their concerns. During this dialogue, be attentive to verbal cues and non-verbal signals, which often reveal significant information about the patient's experience and worries (Cuff, 2020).

Observation of the Patient

Careful observation of the patient begins from the moment they enter the clinical environment. Pay close attention to their body language, facial expressions and the way they walk, as these factors can offer valuable insights into their presenting complaint and overall well-being (Wilson and Childs, 2002). For instance, a patient who limps or frequently shifts their weight may be experiencing musculoskeletal pain, while a lack of eye contact could indicate anxiety or discomfort. Noting how the patient moves from the waiting area to the consultation room – such as hesitancy, guarding a limb or slow movements – may reveal subtle cues about their discomfort, mobility or pain.

During the assessment, it is important to gather information not only from what the patient says but also from their non-verbal signals. Minute details, such as grimacing, rubbing a limb and protective posturing (guarding), should be closely observed since they can provide additional context to the verbal history and help influence further examination (Lamb et al., 2012). Recognising these subtle cues may prompt the clinician to ask targeted questions or perform specific physical examinations, thereby improving diagnostic accuracy and informing the next steps in assessment and management.

Clarify, Repeat and Summarise

Clearly reiterate key information to facilitate understanding of the patient's condition and respond to any questions or concerns (Finucane et al., 2020).

Use Pattern Recognition

Musculoskeletal conditions often follow predictable patterns (GIRFT, 2023; Jones and Lee, 2006). The SOCRATES framework is a good tool for a structured consultation (NICE, 2020; Silverman et al., 2013).

- **Site** – Where is the pain located (area of concern)?
- **Onset** – When did it start (to identify acute/subacute/chronicity)?
- **Character** – How does the pain feel (sharp, dull, burning)?
- **Radiation** – Does the pain spread (to identify referred pattern, if any)?
- **Associated symptoms** – Any additional symptoms (essential to form initial hypothesis)?
- **Timing** – Has it worsened recently (progression of symptoms)?
- **Exacerbating/relieving factors** – What makes it better or worse (facilitates hypothesis, clinical reasoning and management)?
- **Severity** – Pain intensity on a scale of 0–10 (10 being worst pain imagined).

Additional Assessment Components

Assessment Considerations for Younger Patients

In younger patients, MSK presentations are frequently the result of loading, overuse or congenital issues. These individuals are particularly susceptible to conditions such as Osgood Schlatter disease. Osgood Schlatter is a common cause of knee pain in adolescents and arises from repetitive overloading of the patellar tendon. This condition typically manifests during periods of rapid growth, when increased activity levels place additional stress on developing MSK structures (NICE, 2021b).

Assessment Considerations for Middle-aged Patients

In middle-aged individuals, MSK presentations often involve tendon-related changes. These changes are particularly notable in perimenopausal women, in whom hormonal fluctuations play a significant role. During the perimenopausal period, oestrogen levels decrease, which affects tendon resilience. As a result, there is an increased prevalence of gluteal tendinopathies among this demographic. Understanding the influence of hormonal changes on tendon health is essential when assessing and managing MSK complaints in middle-aged patients.

Assessment Considerations for Older Patients

In older adults, MSK complaints are most usually attributed to degenerative changes within the joints and soft tissue structures. Osteoarthritis is a prevalent example, often presenting with symptoms such as joint pain, stiffness and reduced mobility. These deteriorating processes should be carefully considered during the clinical assessment, to understand their impact on function and quality of life (NICE, 2020).

Red Flags in Subjective Assessment

Attention is warranted for patients younger than 20 years and those older than 55, as presentations within these age groups may suggest underlying pathology that necessitates further investigation and a more judicious approach to management.

History of Presenting Condition

It is essential to determine the progression, precipitating factors and any previous occurrences of symptoms, particularly in individuals reporting chronic pain (Irving et al., 2017). The Ideas, Concerns and Expectations (ICE) framework supports patient-centred consultations by systematically addressing patients' beliefs, fears and aspirations regarding their condition (Kurtz et al., 2017). This methodology fosters improved communication, treatment adherence and patient satisfaction by ensuring that management strategies are aligned with patient expectations (Salmon and Young, 2011). For healthcare professionals, ICE contributes to efficient consultations, enhanced rapport and increased diagnostic accuracy through the identification of psychosocial factors affecting symptom presentation (Silverman et al., 2013). In MSK care, where the influence of patient beliefs on affect and recovery is significant, ICE promotes holistic and effective management (Petty, 2011).

Past Medical History and Family History

Employ the mnemonic THREADS to elucidate the way the following conditions impact MSK assessment (Macleod, 2018; Talley and O'Connor, 2021).

- **T**hyroid (hyperthyroidism/hypothyroidism) – Associated muscle pain, fatigue, paraesthesia.
- **H**eart disease – Cardiovascular pathologies associated with chest pain/shoulder pain, fatigue, breathlessness and side-effects of medications resulting in myalgia.
- **R**heumatological conditions – Autoimmune/inflammatory conditions, enthesitis (inflammation of tendon attachments), morning stiffness, muscle and joint aches and pains.
- **E**pilepsy – MSK injuries and side-effects of medications may cause muscle pains and fatigue.
- **A**sthma – Relative contraindication for anti-inflammatory medications.
- **D**iabetes – Associated with shoulder conditions (rotator cuff-related pain syndromes and frozen shoulder), fatigue and myalgia related to medications.
- **S**teroid use – Steroid myopathy and bone density issues (osteopenia/osteoporosis).

Also check for history of any surgeries and fractures to understand their impact on current condition.

Medication History

Identify drug interactions, allergies, sensitivities and contraindications, as well as the use of herbal supplements and over-the-counter medications (NICE, 2018; Stewart, 2005).

Social History

In addition to these medical considerations, understanding a patient's social history is equally important for comprehensive care. The Making Every Contact Count (MECC) approach encourages healthcare professionals to use routine interactions as opportunities to support behaviour change and improve population health, without extending consultation length (Public Health England, 2016). Clinicians can assess these lifestyle factors through targeted questions during patient interviews and signpost or refer as appropriate. Work environment and occupational demands, such as prolonged sedentary postures or manual handling, can influence MSK symptoms. Similarly, activity levels outside work, including sedentary behaviour or high training loads, may affect pain, function and participation. Lifestyle factors such as smoking and alcohol consumption are associated with increased systemic inflammation and impaired tissue healing, while psychological factors can significantly influence pain perception and recovery (Macleod, 2018; Talley and O'Connor, 2021). Recent studies continue to highlight the significant impact of these lifestyle factors on MSK health, highlighting the importance of their assessment and management in clinical practice.

■ Yellow Flags

Yellow flags are psychosocial factors that can increase the risk of chronic pain, disability and poor recovery in MSK conditions (Linton and Shaw, 2011; Nicholas et al., 2011). Unlike red flags, which indicate serious pathology (e.g. fractures, infections, tumours), yellow flags highlight psychological, behavioural and social barriers to recovery (Nicholas et al., 2011).

Categories and Examples of Yellow Flags

Psychological Factors

Psychological yellow flags commonly include fear avoidance behaviours, where individuals avoid movement due to concerns of further injury (for example, believing that moving will cause more harm). Catastrophising thoughts, such as believing one's back is irreparably damaged, and symptoms of depression, anxiety or emotional distress are also prevalent. These factors can significantly exacerbate pain and impede recovery.

Behavioural Factors

Behavioural yellow flags involve passive coping strategies, such as relying on opioids or prolonged bed rest instead of active rehabilitation. Individuals may demonstrate low self-efficacy, doubting their ability to manage pain effectively. Dependence on healthcare providers, indicated by frequent visits, further reflects a passive approach to recovery, which can undermine long-term outcomes.

Social Factors

Social yellow flags are seen in individuals experiencing dissatisfaction at work or high levels of occupational stress. A lack of social support, resulting in feelings of isolation, and issues related to financial compensation – such as extended sick leave or financial crisis – can all contribute to prolonged disability and hinder the rehabilitation process.

Beliefs and Attitudes

Misconceptions regarding diagnosis, such as interpreting back pain as a sign of permanent damage, are important yellow flags. Additionally, a preference for exclusive medical interventions or inconsistent rehabilitation reveals misinformed beliefs and expectations, which may limit engagement with effective recovery strategies.

Clinical Relevance of Yellow Flags

- Individuals presenting multiple yellow flags are at heightened risk for developing chronic pain and persistent disability (Edwards et al., 2016; Foster et al., 2018; Pincus et al., 2002).
- Fear-avoidant behaviours contribute to physical deconditioning and lasting disability (Meinke et al., 2025; Vlaeyen and Linton, 2000).
- Work-related yellow flags may increase the likelihood of extended sick leave and permanent work disability (Jay et al., 2018; Waddell et al., 1993).

Interventions for Yellow Flags in Musculoskeletal Practice

- **Cognitive behavioural therapy (CBT):** Widely recognised as the leading psychological intervention for chronic MSK pain, CBT helps reshape harmful beliefs and lowers disability rates (Gabel et al., 2012; Stearns et al., 2021).
- **Graded exercise therapy (GET):** This supports gradual increases in physical activity, helping to prevent deconditioning and reduce fear avoidance that are major contributors to persistent pain (Gabel et al., 2012; Hockings et al., 2008).
- **Education and reassurance:** Educating patients about pain and reassuring them regarding movement can diminish fear-avoidant behaviours, affirming that activity is safe and encouraging an active approach to recovery over passive management (Gabel et al., 2012; Stearns et al., 2021).
- **Multidisciplinary approach:** Integrating physiotherapy, psychological support and occupational therapy can tackle a broad range of yellow flag issues, such as unsupportive thoughts, emotional challenges and workplace pressures (Gabel et al., 2012; Stearns et al., 2021).

Early Identification and Management of Yellow Flags in Musculoskeletal Practice

Early Identification to Prevent Chronic Disability

Detecting psychosocial 'yellow flags', such as catastrophic thinking and emotional distress, at an early stage is crucial for preventing the development of chronic pain and long-term disability. Prompt recognition allows for timely interventions that can interrupt the progression towards persistent pain and prolonged disability, thereby improving patient outcomes (Gabel et al., 2012; Stearns et al., 2021).

Use of Validated Screening Tools

Validated instruments like the Örebro Musculoskeletal Pain Questionnaire (ÖMPQ) and its modified version (ÖMSQ) are essential for predicting the risk of long-term disability and work absenteeism. Utilising these tools in clinical practice enables practitioners to systematically identify patients who may be vulnerable to chronic MSK pain and related disability (Gabel et al., 2012; Hockings et al., 2008).

Promoting Active Rehabilitation

Active rehabilitation strategies, such as CBT and graded exercise therapy, have demonstrated greater effectiveness in reducing disability and preventing chronicity compared to passive treatments. Encouraging patients to engage in active interventions supports their recovery and helps to minimise the risk of developing persistent pain (Gabel et al., 2012; Stearns et al., 2021).

Addressing Workplace Factors

The Örebro screening tools incorporate work-related questions, allowing clinicians to tailor recommendations for job modifications or graded return-to-work interventions. By considering workplace factors, healthcare providers can better support patients in their recovery and reduce the likelihood of extended absence from work (Stearns et al., 2021).

■ Motivational Interviewing in Musculoskeletal Practice

Role of Motivational Interviewing

Motivational interviewing forms a core component of psychologically informed physiotherapy. By employing this approach, clinicians can help patients to challenge and shift unhelpful pain beliefs, thereby enhancing their willingness to participate in active rehabilitation strategies. This collaborative technique encourages greater patient engagement and can lead to improved outcomes in musculoskeletal care (Stearns et al., 2021).

Applying the PACE Framework

The PACE acronym provides practical guidance for integrating motivational interviewing into brief patient consultations.

- **P – Partnership:** Treat the patient as an equal partner in the conversation, ensuring discussions are collaborative in nature.
- **A – Autonomy, Empathy, Respect and Affirmation:** Foster an environment where the patient's autonomy is valued, and interactions are characterised by empathy, respect and affirmation.
- **C – Compassion:** Support both the physical and psychological aspects of the patient's well-being through compassionate care.
- **E – Evocation:** Motivate the patient to actively participate in developing a plan of action, thereby encouraging self-management and engagement in their rehabilitation journey (Lewin et al., 2001).

Red Flags and Escalation

Indicators of Serious Pathology

Clinicians should remain alert for symptoms and signs that may indicate the presence of a serious underlying pathology. Key red flags include the following.

- Unintentional weight loss exceeding 5% of body weight within the past 6–12 months.
- Progressive symptoms that fail to resolve despite appropriate intervention.
- Pain that is non-mechanical in nature and not associated with movement or specific postures.
- Unremitting night pain that does not improve with repositioning or rest.
- Systemic symptoms such as fever, chills, malaise, fatigue, loss of appetite or night sweats.
- A personal or family history of cancer.
- Recent trauma or fracture.
- Thoracic back pain.
- Age below 20 or above 55 years.
- Recent infection.
- Unexplained swelling or the presence of a mass.
- History of intravenous drug abuse.

If any of these red flags are identified during assessment, the clinician should consider prompt escalation for further medical evaluation (NICE, 2023a). See Figure 1.1.

Clinical Reasoning in Musculoskeletal Practice

Clinical reasoning is fundamental for safe and accurate diagnosis. The process is called hypothetico-deductive reasoning. Clinicians systematically collect the patient's history and interpret presenting symptoms, generating a set of

PATIENT PRESENTS WITH MSK PAIN (ANY REGION)

⇩

Focused history and examination:
- Onset, mechanism of injury
- Location, radiation, pattern of pain
- Impact on function, work, sleep, mood
- Past medical history and medications
- Screen for red flags (trauma, infection, cancer, neuro, vascular)

⇩

ANY RED FLAGS PRESENT?

⇩ YES ⇩

Determine likely serious cause and URGENCY:
- Suspected fracture
- Suspected cauda equina
- Suspected septic arthritis
- Suspected PE/DVT/GCA

⇩

999/ED (e.g. Same-day Urgent suspected cauda equina, urgent cancer pathway, if appropriate)

⇩ NO ⇩

Proceed as non-specific/mechanical/overuse/degenerative MSK pain

⇩

For non-red flag cases:
- Discuss working diagnosis
- Provide education and self-management advice
- Advice to keep active
- Consider simple analgesia as per NICE
- Safety net: tell patient what to watch for and when/how to seek further help
- Plan follow-up/review

Figure 1.1 General MSK assessment and red flag escalation pathway.

initial diagnostic hypotheses (Norman, 2005). As the consultation progresses and more information is gathered through examination and discussion, these hypotheses are rigorously tested, refined or discarded. This iterative approach allows the clinician to move from a broad range of differential diagnoses towards a more focused conclusion that is supported by evidence (Eva, 2005). In tandem with this analytical method, pattern recognition plays a significant role. This process entails the clinician's intuitive alignment of the patient's presenting characteristics with previously encountered 'illness scripts', thereby facilitating efficient diagnostic reasoning (Norman, 2005).

Furthermore, effective clinical reasoning relies on metacognition. This is the ability to reflect on one's own thought processes, identify potential cognitive biases and monitor the accuracy of both pattern recognition and hypothesis testing (Croskerry, 2009). Through metacognitive awareness, clinicians can ensure that their reasoning remains robust and justified. By integrating narrative reasoning, clinical knowledge, hypothesis formation and ongoing self-reflection, clinicians can reach diagnostic decisions that are both safe and evidence based. This comprehensive approach highlights sound clinical judgement in musculoskeletal assessment.

Objective Examination

The objective examination in musculoskeletal assessment is systematic and thorough. It should include evaluating the joint immediately above and below the area of concern to identify whether symptoms may be correlated or referred. Joint movements should be assessed to detect any restrictions or abnormal patterns. Additionally, the strength of muscles responsible for movement at the affected region is tested.

Functional patterns are also observed, particularly in the assessment of lower body joints. This involves evaluating the patient's ability to stand, sit, squat and perform single leg balancing, thereby gaining insight into how symptoms influence their daily activities. This structured approach ensures that both local and neighbouring structures are assessed, helping to clarify the diagnosis by linking observed functional limitations to specific anatomical findings (NICE, 2022a).

Inspection

During the inspection phase, the clinician should carefully observe for any signs of asymmetry (e.g. scoliosis), changes in skin colour (e.g. redness, pallor, bruises), muscle wasting, swelling, lumps/bumps, obvious deformity (valgus/varus in knee) or any other anatomical deviations. These visual assessments help to identify external indications of underlying MSK conditions (Turnpenney et al., 2015).

Palpation

The palpation component involves feeling for differences in tissue temperature, detecting muscle spasms and identifying areas of tenderness. These findings can provide important information regarding inflammation, structures involved or localised pain (Salisbury et al., 2022a).

Testing Procedures

- **Range of motion (ROM):** The range of motion is assessed through both active and passive movements. Active movement requires the patient to voluntarily move the joint through actions such as flexion, extension, rotation and lateral flexion. Passive movement is carried out by the examiner, moving the joint without the patient's assistance to identify any restrictions or abnormal patterns (McCormick et al., 2020).
- **Resisted tests:** The patient performs a movement against resistance applied by the examiner. This helps evaluate muscle strength and presence of any pain during resistance (Wilson and Childs, 2002).
- **Functional tests:** Functional assessments involve asking the patient to carry out activities relevant to their daily life or occupation. For example, a builder performs a squat to lift bricks, thereby representing activities at work. The clinician should also assess activities of daily living (ADLs), such as sitting, standing and driving, and document any limitations observed (GIRFT, 2023).
- **Special tests:** These are specific, validated procedures designed to confirm or rule out joint conditions or pathologies. The reliability of these tests is established through research and clinical practice (Cuff, 2020).

Neurological Integrity

Evaluating neurological integrity is essential when nerve or central nervous system compression is suspected. Assessment should include reflexes, dermatomes, myotomes, balance, gait, co-ordination, Babinski, clonus and cranial nerve exams as and when indicated. These findings are fundamental for comprehensive MSK evaluation (Vilgran et al., 2023).

Gut Feeling in Musculoskeletal Practice

Gut feeling in clinical practice has been described as an intuitive sense that something is wrong, even when the clinician cannot fully articulate the reason (Elstein et al., 1978; Norman, 2005). This intuitive response often presents as a sense that clinical information does not fully align, or that the overall picture feels incongruent with typical patterns (Norman, 2005). Recognising and appropriately responding to gut feeling is part of safe, evidence-based clinical reasoning (Finucane et al., 2020; Jones and Lee, 2006).

Key elements include the following.

- **Effective communication** – Clarify the concerns with the patient and ensure their narrative is fully explored (Kurtz et al., 2017).
- **Listening actively** – Patients may reveal subtle cues or inconsistencies that trigger intuitive concern (Silverman et al., 2013).
- **Using the clinical reasoning process** – Integrate subjective and objective findings; identify gaps or mismatches (Elstein et al., 1978; Jones and Lee, 2006).
- **Acknowledging discordant information** – A sense that 'something does not fit the pattern' should prompt further exploration (Norman, 2005).
- **Articulating the concern** – Ask yourself, 'What makes me think something is not right?' (Croskerry, 2009).
- **Recognising self-cues** – Clinicians often describe a 'lurch in the stomach' or 'alarm bells', signalling heightened alertness and the need for further assessment or safety netting (Croskerry, 2009; Finucane et al., 2020).

These intuitive cues should not replace objective assessment but may act as powerful early warning signals, prompting reflective practice, further questioning, closer follow-up or appropriate escalation to ensure patient safety (Elstein et al., 1978; Finucane et al., 2020; NICE, 2016d).

Patient Education

It is important to use simple language and relatable examples when discussing conditions, ensuring the patient can easily grasp the key concepts involved (Freeman et al., 2002). To further support comprehension, clinicians should incorporate visual aids and online resources where appropriate. These tools can help illustrate complex ideas and provide additional reference material for patients to review at their own pace considering their health literacy level (Cuff, 2020). When delivering information, applying the 'chunk and check' method is beneficial. This involves breaking information into smaller, manageable sections and pausing to confirm the patient's understanding before moving on. The 'teach back' technique can be used to check understanding, where the patient is asked to repeat the information in their own words, ensuring clarity and retention of key messages (NICE, 2021a).

Management Options and Planning for Recovery

Evidence-based Management Approaches

Musculoskeletal management utilises evidence-based treatment approaches as outlined in established guidelines (NICE, 2016a). Incorporating these recommendations ensures that the care provided aligns with current best practice and optimises patient outcomes.

Decision-making tools should be employed to inform patients and support a shared decision-making process. These tools are available for a range of conditions, including carpal tunnel syndrome, hip and knee osteoarthritis, Dupuytren's contracture and chronic pain, and can help both clinicians and patients navigate complex treatment choices (Personalised Care Institute, 2020b). Clinicians should refer to guidance from NICE and the Getting It Right First Time (GIRFT) programme, which provides comprehensive, evidence-based recommendations to support clinical decisions (GIRFT, 2023). For analgesia options, consideration of the World Health Organization's pain ladder is recommended to ensure appropriate selection and escalation of pain management strategies (WHO, 1986).

Planning Recovery and Follow-up

Setting realistic expectations regarding recovery is a crucial element in effective management. Patients benefit from clear advice about the typical healing times for affected structures; for example, soft tissues generally require approximately 16–18 weeks to heal. Explaining this anticipated timeline enables patients to understand when it is appropriate to begin loading, rehabilitating and pacing their activities throughout the recovery process (Wilson and Childs, 2002).

To ensure that patients can access important information as needed, clinicians should offer clear safety-netting advice. This may be supported with written materials, emails or messages, so that patients have guidance readily available if concerns arise or their condition changes (Siddiqui et al., 2020). Outline and discuss the next steps in the management plan with the patient. This collaborative approach enhances patient compliance, fosters trust and encourages adherence to the interventions that have been recommended (Turnpenney et al., 2015).

Time Management in Primary Care

In the primary care environment, clinicians are frequently confronted with notable time pressures and an ever-increasing workload. Standard consultations allow a maximum of 10 minutes, which necessitates a highly structured approach to both patient assessment and questioning. Within this limited timeframe, it is critical for healthcare professionals to employ well-organised and targeted strategies to maximise the quality of care provided.

Competent assessment techniques are vital for ensuring that all pertinent aspects of a patient's history and examination are efficiently addressed. By utilising structured questioning methods, clinicians can gather comprehensive information systematically. This approach enables them to swiftly and accurately identify key health concerns, ensuring that no important details are overlooked during the consultation.

Implementing these focused strategies allows practitioners to deliver thorough and effective care, even when operating within the constraints of brief appointments. By maintaining such standards, clinicians can ensure high-quality patient interactions despite the demands of a busy practice.

This text provides practical guidance for conducting complete and careful assessments in primary care settings with short appointment durations. By adhering to these methods, primary care professionals can optimise patient outcomes and enhance the overall quality of their consultations elaborated in the MSK consultation pathway (Figure 1.2).

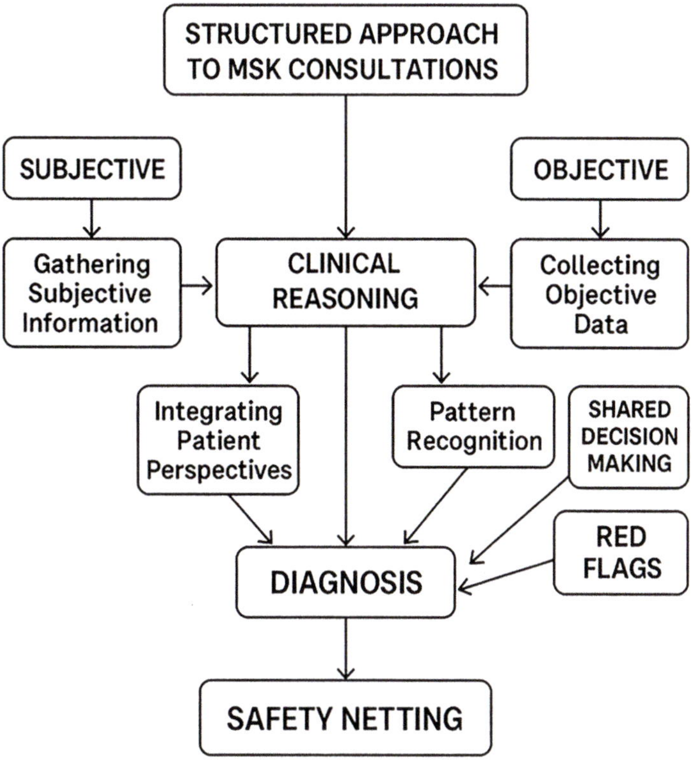

Figure 1.2 Musculoskeletal consultation pathway.

CHAPTER 2

Red Flags and Visceral Masqueraders

Introduction to Red Flags

Red flags are clinical indicators that suggest the presence of a potentially serious condition rather than a straightforward musculoskeletal disorder. According to NICE (2022a), which provides national clinical guidelines for primary care practitioners, recognising these signs is essential to inpatient assessment to help clinicians differentiate between benign and life-threatening conditions (Finucane et al., 2020).

Given the small but substantial proportion of serious cases, it is important to understand which conditions may present as red flags. These include malignancies such as metastatic cancer and multiple myeloma, infections like osteomyelitis and discitis, and neurological emergencies including cauda equina syndrome (Jones and Lee, 2006). In addition, vascular emergencies, such as deep vein thrombosis (DVT) and aortic aneurysm, demand immediate assessment due to their potentially life-threatening consequences (Finucane et al., 2020). Fractures, encompassing both osteoporotic and occult, also require urgent imaging and intervention to prevent further complications (Dijkstra et al., 2020).

Although the majority of MSK presentations are benign, literature reports that approximately 1% of all MSK cases in primary care involve serious underlying pathology (NICE, 2020).

NICE (2020) is considered the gold standard for epidemiological data and best practices in UK primary care, further highlighting the necessity for thorough clinical evaluation to promptly recognise and address these critical cases.

The ability to recognise red flags without delay is vital. Prompt identification and action are essential to avoid diagnostic delays and ensure that patients receive timely and appropriate intervention, emphasising the importance of early intervention to improve patient outcomes (Bennett et al., 2016).

To systematically incorporate red flag screening into routine assessments, clinicians should adopt a step-by-step approach. Each MSK evaluation should begin with targeted questions related to recent trauma, unexplained weight loss, fever or neurological symptoms. Clinicians may use a structured checklist to ensure no key indicators are missed. If any red flag is identified, immediate referral or further investigation is warranted. This methodical approach enables practitioners to efficiently identify serious pathologies and safety net patients, ensuring patient safety and optimal care. A summary of red flags is captured in (Table 2.1).

Table 2.1 Red flags summary.

Red flag domain	Examples	Possible serious pathology	Action (NICE-aligned)
Constitutional	Unexplained weight loss, night sweats, fever, general malaise	Malignancy, infection, systemic disease	Urgent GP/medical review; bloods; consider urgent imaging
Neurological	Progressive limb weakness, saddle anaesthesia, bowel/bladder dysfunction, gait disturbance, sexual dysfunction	Cauda equina, spinal cord compression, myelopathy	Same-day urgent referral to ED/spinal service (NG59)
Trauma	Major trauma, high-impact injury, inability to bear weight, deformity	Fracture, dislocation, internal injury	ED assessment, imaging as per NG37/NG38
Infection risk	Fever + joint pain, recent surgery or injection, IVDU, immunosuppression	Septic arthritis, osteomyelitis, discitis	Urgent same-day assessment and labs/imaging.
Vascular	Pale/cool limb, pulselessness, severe calf pain/swelling, chest pain/SOB	Acute limb ischemia, DVT/PE, ACS	999/urgent ED depending on presentation
Cancer history	New bone pain, night pain, unexplained persistent pain in someone with cancer history	Bone metastasis, primary bone malignancy	Urgent suspected cancer pathway

Red flag domain	Examples	Possible serious pathology	Action (NICE-aligned)
Inflammatory	Prolonged morning stiffness, multiple swollen joints, visual symptoms, jaw claudication	RA, axial SpA, PMR, GCA	Rapid rheumatology/ medical referral as per NG100/NG65 and CKS PMR/GCA

Abbreviations: ACS, Acute Coronary Syndrome; CKS, Clinical Knowledge Summaries; DVT, Deep Vein Thrombosis; ED, Emergency Department; GCA, Giant Cell Arteritis; IVDU, Intravenous Drug Use; PE, Pulmonary Embolism; PMR, Polymyalgia Rheumatica; RA, Rheumatoid Arthritis; SOB, Shortness of Breath; SpA, Spondyloarthropathy.

Upper Limb Red Flags

Certain conditions affecting the shoulder, elbow, wrist and hand may mimic MSK issues but can indicate serious pathology (Academy of Physical Medicine, 2018).

- **Pancoast tumour (lung cancer at apex):** Shoulder pain, arm pain, muscle wasting and Horner's syndrome (ptosis = drooping of the eyelid, anhidrosis = loss of sweating function on the face, miosis = constricted pupil) may indicate a malignancy requiring urgent chest X-ray and referral via urgent suspected cancer pathway (Vilgran et al., 2023).
- **Trauma/fracture:** Sudden, acute trauma in upper limb due to osteoporosis, fall, osteomyelitis (bone infection), etc.; escalate to emergency immediately (Finucane et al., 2020).
- **Inflammatory/autoimmune pathologies:** Polymyalgia rheumatica (PMR) (pain in shoulder girdle and hips with fatigue, morning stiffness, fever, weight loss), inflammatory arthropathy (females are more prone to cervical and thoracic pains related to inflammatory arthritis), rheumatoid arthritis (shoulder osteoarthritis is commonly associated with rheumatoid arthritis) that causes pain, stiffness and inflammation – urgent referral to rheumatology is warranted (Finucane et al., 2020).
- **Osteosarcoma/Ewing's sarcoma:** Although more commonly affecting the pelvis and lower limbs, progressive pain, night pain, swelling and weight loss suggest possible bone cancer, demanding MRI and urgent orthopaedic referral (Ng and Chan, 2024).
- **Septic arthritis:** A hot, swollen joint with fever/chills and severe pain may indicate a joint infection requiring urgent blood tests, joint aspiration and referral to emergency (Stewart, 2005).
- **Avascular necrosis (AVN) upper limb:** Progressive pain with a history of steroid use/alcoholism/trauma requires X-ray to confirm and onward orthopaedic referral is warranted (Turnpenney et al., 2015).
- **Special considerations for shoulder pain:** Shoulder pain with a missed menstrual period could indicate an ectopic pregnancy (Silverman et al., 2013).

- **DVT (upper limb):** The presence of redness, swelling, characterised by Urschel's sign (dilated veins in upper limb), and pain in the upper limb should prompt a Doppler ultrasound and D-dimer blood test to evaluate for venous thrombosis. Although rare, this condition can lead to severe outcomes, particularly following recent surgery or trauma. Sudden-onset shoulder pain post-surgery might indicate a pulmonary embolism or DVT (NICE, 2023b).

Lower Limb Red Flags

Certain lower limb conditions require urgent assessment and referral due to their potential for serious morbidity or mortality (Elstein et al., 1978).

- **Lower limb cancers** can present with fever/chills, night sweats, unremitting night pains, malaise, loss of appetite, unintentional weight loss of >5% of body weight in 6–12 months and the following specific symptoms.
  - Osteoid osteoma: Young adults with severe hip pains worse at night, better with activity, associated with cancer red flags may indicate bone cancer.
  - Aneurysm/colorectal cancer: Hip/groin pain with alternating abdominal pains.
  - Testicular cancer: Hip/groin pain of insidious onset especially males between the age of 18 and 24 associated with cancer red flags.
  - Extremity cancers: Bone pain, antalgic gait, constant night pains, vaginal/penile discharge, lymphadenopathy associated with cancer red flags (Finucane et al., 2020).
- **Stress fracture of femur:** Aching deep pain, worse with activity better with rest and limited hip abduction, urgent fracture clinic referral is warranted (Finucane et al., 2020).
- **Lower limb fractures (osteoporotic or pathological):** Inability to bear weight with an externally rotated or shortened leg suggests the possibility of fracture in the hip, requiring urgent orthopaedic assessment (Lamb et al., 2012).
- **Septic arthritis (hip/knee/ankle):** A red, swollen joint with fever/chills and severe pain requires urgent IV antibiotics and emergency referral (Wilson and Childs, 2002).
- **Avascular necrosis (AVN) hip, navicular, cuboid:** Progressive pain with a history of steroid use/alcoholism/trauma requires X-ray to confirm and if an intervention is planned post X-ray it requires an MRI (Turnpenney et al., 2015).
- **Deep vein thrombosis (DVT):** Unilateral limb swelling, redness, pain, warmth, positive Homan's sign in calf (painful dorsiflexion of foot in extended knee position) warrant Doppler ultrasound, D-dimer blood test and anticoagulation therapy. In clinic complete Well's criteria for escalation to emergency (Dijkstra et al., 2020).

- **Compartment syndrome:** Severe limb pain with pallor, paraesthesia, pulselessness and paralysis (4Ps) is a surgical emergency requiring immediate intervention (BOA, 2022).
- **Inflammatory/autoimmune pathologies:** Polymyalgia rheumatica (PMR) (pain in shoulder girdle and hips with fatigue, morning stiffness, fever, weight loss), inflammatory arthropathy (females are more prone to enthesitis – Achilles and plantar fascia being the most common areas), rheumatoid arthritis (hip and knee osteoarthritis are commonly associated with rheumatoid arthritis); urgent referral to rheumatology is warranted (Finucane et al., 2020).

Visceral Masqueraders: When Musculoskeletal Pain is Not Musculoskeletal

Many serious visceral conditions mimic MSK pain, leading to misdiagnosis. It is crucial to differentiate true MSK disorders from systemic pathologies (NICE, 2022a). Common visceral masqueraders include the following.

- **Abdominal aortic aneurysm (AAA):** Lower back or hip pain with a pulsatile abdominal mass, cardiovascular risk factors and blood pressure changes may indicate an aortic aneurysm requiring X-ray to measure the size; if aorta is >80 mm there is a greater than 50% chance of rupture. Assess lumbar spine, lower limb neurological and vascular examination – if exam indicates vascular pathology on contrary to musculoskeletal, referral for urgent abdominal ultrasound is recommended and plan referral to vascular team (Salisbury et al., 2022b).
- **Multiple myeloma:** Unexplained back pain with bony tenderness, fever/chills, unexplained weight loss >5% of body weight in the past 6–12 months, loss of appetite, fatigue, malaise, unremitting night pains and anaemia could be an early sign of malignancy. **CRAB** mnemonic represents hyper**c**alcaemia, **R**enal failure, **A**naemia and **B**one lesion, which are diagnostic criteria for myeloma. Urgent blood tests – full blood count (FBC), bone profile, kidney (U/E), serum immunoglobins, urine Bence Jones proteins and MRI are gold standard investigations via urgent suspected cancer pathway (Stewart, 2005).
- **Visceral referred pain:** Cardiac, gastrointestinal and pulmonary conditions can present as shoulder or back pain, requiring thorough systemic assessment (Elstein et al., 1978).

Key Takeaways

Red Flags in Musculoskeletal Assessment

Red flags serve as essential warning signs that may indicate the presence of severe underlying conditions, necessitating prompt and decisive intervention (Dijkstra et al., 2020).

Upper Limb Red Flags

In the evaluation of upper limb symptoms, it is vital to remain alert for red flags such as suspected malignancies, vascular disorders and AVN. These conditions can present subtly but may rapidly progress if not identified and managed early (Academy of Physical Medicine, 2018).

Lower Limb Red Flags

Red flags within the lower limb include the possibility of fractures, acute vascular emergencies and infections. These presentations require urgent recognition to prevent long-term morbidity (Bennett et al., 2016).

Visceral Masqueraders

It is important to recognise that visceral conditions can mimic MSK pain. Careful clinical judgement is required to distinguish these cases from mechanical or MSK causes, as visceral conditions may be life-threatening if unnoticed (NICE, 2023b).

Urgency of Referral and Imaging

Whenever red flags are suspected during assessment, urgent referral to the appropriate specialist and prompt imaging are warranted. The early identification of these warning signs is crucial in ensuring timely intervention and improving patient outcomes (Finucane et al., 2020).

CHAPTER **2a**

Spinal Red Flags

Introduction

Spinal red flags are clinical indicators that suggest the presence of serious underlying pathology, including fractures, infections, malignancy or neurological compromise. Recognising these warning signs is vital, as failure to do so may result in permanent disability or even life-threatening complications (NICE, 2023b).

Although serious spinal conditions account for only about 1% of all musculoskeletal (MSK) presentations, their potential severity necessitates a meticulous and thorough assessment pathway (Figure 2a.1) (Finucane et al., 2020). The main spinal red flags, along with their associated symptoms, are summarised in Table 2a.1.

Table 2a.1 Key spinal red flags and associated conditions.

Red flag	Potential serious condition	Next steps
Age >50 or <20 years	Malignancy, infection	Imaging (X-ray, request MRI via emergency referral) if persistent pain (Goubran and Tomlinson, 2023)
Progressive, unremitting pain	Spinal tumour, infection	Urgent request for MRI via emergency and blood tests (Finucane et al., 2020)
Severe thoracic pain	Malignancy, vertebral fracture	Request MRI via orthopaedic referral for high-risk patients (Finucane et al., 2020)

(Continued)

Table 2a.1 *(Continued)*

Red flag	**Potential serious condition**	**Next steps**
History of cancer	Metastatic spinal cord compression (MSCC)	Request MRI via urgent suspected cancer pathway referral or MSCC co-ordinator (NICE, 2023b)
Unexplained weight loss, night sweats	Malignancy, systemic infection	Blood tests, urgent request for MRI via urgent suspected cancer pathway referral (Turnpenney et al., 2015)
Saddle anaesthesia, urinary overflow incontinence, sexual dysfunction, bilateral paraesthesia, bowel incontinence, flaccid anus	Cauda equina syndrome (CES)	Request MRI via emergency referral followed by neurosurgery referral (GIRFT, 2023)
Severe lumbar pain + pulsatile abdominal mass	Abdominal aortic aneurysm (AAA)	Urgent abdominal ultrasound and urgent vascular referral

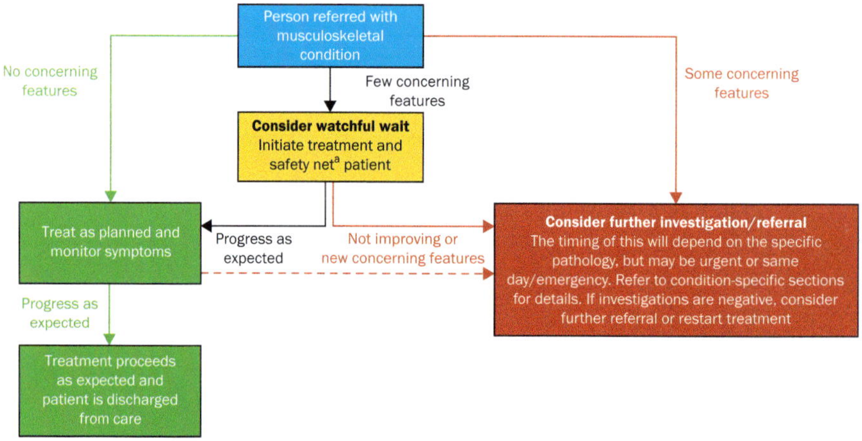

Figure 2a.1 Spinal red flags pathway (Finucane et al., 2020).

Emergency Spinal Conditions

Cauda Equina Syndrome

Cauda equina syndrome (CES) is a surgical emergency which affects 1–3/100,000 in England (Swadling et al., 2024). An anatomical representation of the spinal cord and the cauda equina can be seen in Figure 2a.2, with stages of CES.

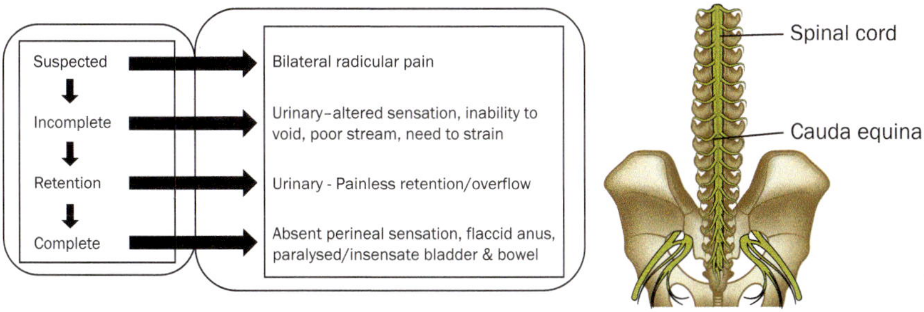

Figure 2a.2 Cauda equina: anatomical illustration and stages of CES.

Compression of the cauda equina nerve roots can lead to permanent neurological damage.

Red Flag Symptoms

- Bilateral paraesthesia, perianal numbness, saddle anaesthesia,
- Bladder dysfunction (urinary retention/incontinence, voiding issues), bowel incontinence.
- Sensory/motor weakness deficits, loss of anal tone (NICE, 2023b).
- Sexual dysfunction – inability to achieve erection or ejaculation in males and inability to achieve orgasm or lack of sensation/feeling during sex in females.

Management

- Urgent emergency referral from primary care following the GIRFT pathway; include examination questions.
- Immediate MRI in secondary care.
- Neurosurgical decompression within 48 hours (GIRFT, 2023).

Figure 2a.3 illustrates an emergency card created by the Musculoskeletal Association of Chartered Physiotherapists (MACP) given to suspected cauda equina patients for safety netting (MACP, 2016).

Cauda Equina Syndrome Warning Signs

- Loss of feeling/pins and needles between your inner thighs or genitals
- Numbness in or around your back passage or buttocks
- Altered feeling when using toilet paper to wipe yourself
- Increasing difficulty when you try to urinate
- Increasing difficulty when you try to stop or control your flow of urine
- Loss of sensation when you pass urine
- Leaking urine or recent need to use pads
- Not knowing when your bladder is either full or empty
- Inability to stop a bowel movement or leaking
- Loss of sensation when you pass a bowel motion
- Change in ability to achieve an erection or ejaculate
- Loss of sensation in genitals during sexual intercourse

Any combination seek help immediately

Figure 2a.3 MACP card for patient safety netting.

Metastatic Spinal Cord Compression

An oncological emergency, MSCC, occurs in 5–10% of cancer patients, leading to irreversible paralysis if untreated (Salisbury et al., 2022b).

Red Flag Symptoms

- New-onset back pain in cancer patients.
- Pain worse when lying down, unremitting night pain.
- Limb weakness, sensory loss, bladder/bowel dysfunction.

Management

- In primary care, refer onwards.
- Urgent MRI within 24 hours in secondary care as per guidelines (GIRFT, 2023).
- Emergency MSCC co-ordinator if known and neurosurgical referral (McCormick et al., 2020).

Figure 2.4a illustrates a Metastatic cord compression (MSCC) card for safety netting.

Metastatic spinal cord compression

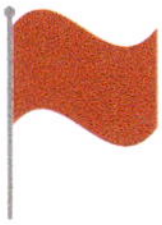

Past medical history of cancer

Early diagnosis is essential

Combination of red flags increases suspicion

Early warning signs of MSCC

R- Referred back pain is multisegmental/band like

E- Escalating pain which is poorly responsive to treatment

D- Different character or site to previous symptoms

F- Funny feelings, odd sensation or heavy legs

L- Lying flat increases back pain

A- Agonising pain causing anguish and despair

G- Gait disturbance, unsteadiness, especially on stairs

S- Sleep grossly disturbed due to pain being worse at night

Established motor/sensory/bladder/bowel disturbances- late signs

Figure 2a.4 Metastatic cord compression (MSCC) card for safety netting (Christie NHS Foundation Trust, 2016).

Spinal Infections – Serious Masqueraders

Spinal infections can mimic mechanical back pain, delaying diagnosis (Finucane et al., 2020).

Common causes include *Staphylococcus aureus* (50–60% of cases) and tuberculosis (Pott's disease). Risk factors include immunosuppression, IV drug use, recent surgery (Goubran and Tomlinson, 2023).

Red Flag Symptoms

- Severe, persistent back pain, fever, night sweats.
- Neurological deterioration (limb weakness, incontinence).
- Pain worsening despite conventional treatment (Salisbury et al., 2022b).

Management

- In primary care, refer onwards to secondary care/orthopaedic referral.
- In secondary care, MRI (gold standard) and intravenous antibiotics, neurosurgical evaluation if epidural abscess is present (NICE, 2023b).

Spinal Fractures – High Risk in Trauma and Osteoporosis

Up to 70% of vertebral fractures go undiagnosed due to misinterpretation as mechanical back pain. Common areas of fracture are shown in Figure 2a.5 (Royal Osteoporosis Society, 2022).

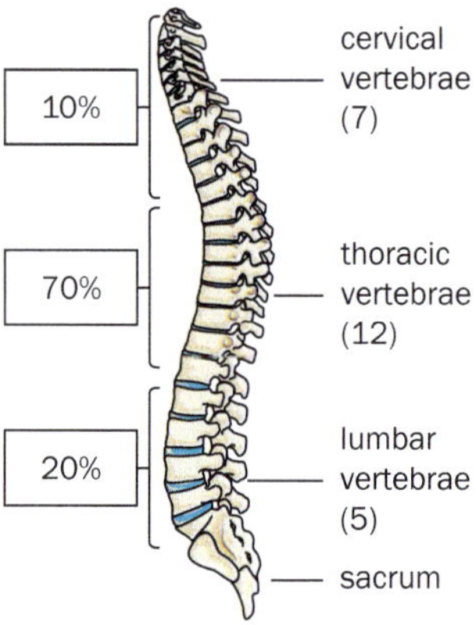

Figure 2a.5 Common areas of spinal fracture.

Common causes include the following (McCormick et al., 2020).

- High-energy trauma (falls, accidents).
- Osteoporotic compression fractures (low-energy trauma in older people).
- Crohn's/poor absorption issues due to long-term intake of omeprazole.
- Eating disorders.
- Medicines: Corticosteroid >3 months 5–7.5 mg/day.
- Rheumatoid arthritis.
- Habits: Alcohol >3 units/day, smoking >30/day.
- Pathological fractures: Malignancy/infection/space-occupying lesion.

Red flag symptoms include:

- Acute, severe back pain, worsened by movement or weight bearing.
- Vertebral tenderness on palpation – percussion test.
- Neurological symptoms suggest spinal cord involvement.

Management

- First-line investigation – urgent X-ray in primary care.
- In secondary care:

  - MRI if neurological symptoms or malignancy is suspected.
  - Prescription of bisphosphonates for osteoporosis-related fractures in primary/secondary care (Royal Osteoporosis Society, 2022).
  - Spinal fusion or vertebroplasty for unstable fractures, via spinal pathway referral.

Abdominal Aortic Aneurysm – Vascular Masquerader

Abdominal aortic aneurysm rupture has a 90% mortality rate if untreated (McCormick et al., 2020).

Red flag symptoms include:

- Severe lumbar/flank pain, radiating to the groin.
- Pulsatile abdominal mass, hypotension, syncope.
- History of smoking, hypertension, atherosclerosis (Goubran and Tomlinson, 2023).

Management

- First line of management in primary care – urgent abdominal ultrasound.
- Management in secondary care:
  - Emergency ultrasound or CT angiography.
  - Urgent vascular referral for aneurysms >5.5 cm of aorta (NICE, 2023b).

Key Takeaways

Serious Pathologies in Musculoskeletal Presentations

Approximately 1% of MSK cases are due to serious underlying pathology. For this reason, it is crucial to assess for red flag symptoms in all patients presenting with back pain or related MSK complaints (Finucane et al., 2020).

Cauda Equina Syndrome

Cauda equina syndrome is a medical emergency that necessitates immediate referral for emergency MRI and surgical decompression. Intervention should occur within 48 hours to reduce the risk of permanent disability (GIRFT, 2023).

Metastatic Spinal Cord Compression

Metastatic spinal cord compression is considered an oncological emergency. Prompt recognition and urgent referral to specialist services are essential to prevent irreversible neurological damage (Salisbury et al., 2022a).

Spinal Infections

Spinal infections can closely resemble mechanical back pain. However, the presence of fever, neurological deficits or worsening pain should raise suspicion and prompt urgent MRI imaging to confirm the diagnosis (NICE, 2023b).

Osteoporotic Vertebral Fractures

Osteoporotic fractures occur commonly in older patients. The sudden onset of pain following minor trauma should prompt imaging, such as an X-ray, in a primary care setting.

Pain that is aggravated by weight bearing and relieved by non-weight-bearing postures is suggestive of such fractures (Royal Osteoporosis Society, 2022).

Abdominal Aortic Aneurysm

Abdominal aortic aneurysm should be suspected in patients presenting with severe back pain and vascular risk factors. Rupture is often fatal without immediate intervention. Additional signs, such as bruising on the abdomen (Cullen sign or Grey Turner sign), are indicative of rupture and warrant urgent medical attention.

CHAPTER 3

The Cervical Spine

Introduction

Neck pain is common. Up to 70% of people will experience it at some point in life, and 43% of UK adults report chronic neck pain which results in major work absence and economic burden (NICE, 2023c). The cervical spine is essential for maintaining head support, safeguarding the spinal cord and enabling a wide range of movements. Its anatomical intricacy, combined with its proximity to both neurological and vascular structures, means that disorders of the cervical region can manifest in various ways. These manifestations may range from mechanical pain to significant neurological impairments, emphasising the importance of careful evaluation (Bogduk, 2012; NICE, 2023c).

This chapter outlines a systematic approach to the assessment of the cervical spine. It covers common cervical spine conditions (Table 3.1), highlights red flag symptoms necessitating urgent intervention (Table 3.2), special tests for pathologies (Table 3.3), summarises conditions (Table 3.4) and evidence-based management strategies to guide clinical practice (Childs et al., 2008). Figure 3.1 shows cervical spine anatomy.

Anatomy Overview

The cervical spine consists of:

- **Seven vertebrae (C1–C7):** Providing stability and mobility.
- **Intervertebral discs:** Absorbing shock and allowing movement.
- **Ligaments and muscles:** Ensuring structural support.
- **Cervical nerve roots (C1–T1):** Controlling upper limb function (Standring, 2021), as shown in Figure 3.1.

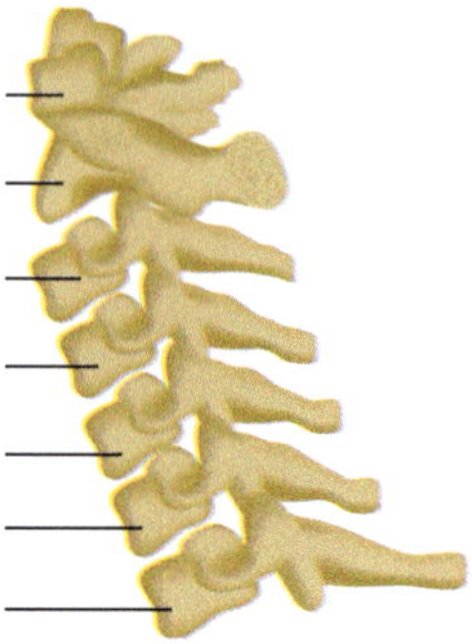

Figure 3.1 Cervical spine anatomy.

Table 3.1 Common cervical spine conditions.

Condition	Cause	Symptoms	Age group	Investigations	Management
Mechanical neck pain	Overuse, poor posture, stress Any age M=F	Localised pain, stiffness, referred headache	Any age, common in middle-aged adults	Routine X-ray in primary care/MRI only if persistent to rule out sinister pathologies via secondary care referral	Referral to physiotherapy, ergonomic adjustments, NSAIDs* (Bronfort et al., 2016)
Cervical disc herniation	Disc degeneration, trauma, overuse M=F	Neck pain, radicular symptoms (arm pain, weakness, numbness)	Varied age	MRI is the gold standard via secondary care referral	Referral to physiotherapy, NSAIDs*, nerve pain medication, possible surgical referral (Jensen et al., 2022)
Cervical stenosis	Degenerative disc disease, osteophytes, narrowed spinal canal >40	Progressive neck pain, bilateral arm symptoms, weakness/ atrophy	Middle-aged to elderly	MRI gold standard via secondary care referral	Referral to physiotherapy, pain management, surgery if severe (Nouri et al., 2015)

Condition	Cause	Symptoms	Age group	Investigations	Management
Whiplash-associated disorder	Trauma (e.g. motor vehicle collisions)	Neck stiffness, headaches, dizziness, vision changes, psychological symptoms, etc.	Any age	X-ray in emergency/ MRI if unresolved symptoms via secondary care referral	Referral to physiotherapy, graded exercise therapy, psychosocial support (Carroll et al., 2009)
Cervicogenic headache	Dysfunction of upper cervical joints/soft tissues	Unilateral headache triggered by neck movement	Middle-aged adults	Symptom-based diagnosis	Referral to physiotherapy, manual therapy, ergonomic modifications (Hall et al., 2010)

*NSAIDs – if allowed and tolerated or start with paracetamol.

Abbreviations: MRI, magnetic resonance imaging; NSAID, non-steroidal anti-inflammatory drug.

Red Flags in Cervical Spine Disorders

Screening for Cervical Arterial Dysfunction

- **5 Ds:** Diplopia (double vision), dysphagia (difficulty swallowing), dysarthria (difficulty in speech), drop attacks (uncontrolled falls), dizziness (room or patient spinning).
- **3 Ns:** Numbness, nystagmus, nausea (Thomas et al., 2019).

Other Neurological Warning Signs

- **Ataxia, weakness, dropping objects, muscle atrophy**: Suggests cervical **myelopathy** (Nouri et al., 2015).
- **Radicular pain (C5–T1), reflex changes, myotome weakness and sensory changes**: Indicates cervical **radiculopathy** (Childs et al., 2008).

Table 3.2 Cervical spine red flags and emergency referral criteria.

Red flag	Potential serious condition	Immediate action
Bilateral neurological deficits	Cervical myelopathy	Referral to secondary care. Urgent MRI, neurosurgery referral (Nouri et al., 2015)

(Continued)

Table 3.2 (*Continued*)

Red flag	Potential serious condition	Immediate action
Severe, persistent neck pain unrelieved by rest	Infection, malignancy	Urgent blood tests. Referral to secondary care – MRI (NICE, 2023a)
Progressive weakness, hyper-reflexia, spasticity	Cervical cord compression	Referral to secondary care. Neurology/neurosurgery referral (Childs et al., 2008)
Acute-onset neck pain with fever, malaise	Meningitis, spinal infection	Emergency referral (Standring, 2021)
Major trauma (fall, car accident, high-impact injury)	Cervical fracture/ dislocation	Immobilisation, emergency X-ray or CT referral via secondary care imaging or fracture clinic (Bogduk, 2012)

Abbreviations: CT, computed tomography; MRI, magnetic resonance imaging.

Cervical Spine Assessment Protocol

Observation

- Assess skin colour, swelling, lumps/bumps, muscle wasting.
- Look for spasms, asymmetry or involuntary movements (Jensen et al., 2022).

Palpation

- Check for tenderness, muscle tension, ligament sprains (Hall et al., 2010).

Range of Motion Testing

- Assess flexion, extension, rotation, side flexion.
- Painful movements suggest joint dysfunction or soft tissue injury (Carroll et al., 2009).

Neurological Examination

- **Dermatomes (C3–T1)**: Sensory testing.
- **Myotomes**: Motor strength assessment (Figure 3.2).
- **Reflexes:** Biceps (C5–C6), triceps (C7), brachioradialis (C6) (Nouri et al., 2015).
- **Cranial nerve tests** for facial sensory changes.
- **Babinski and clonus** for upper motor neuron changes.

C1, C2	Cervical flexion
C3	Cervical side flexion
C4	Scapula elevation
C5	Shoulder abduction
C6	Elbow flexion and wrist extension
C7	Elbow extension and wrist flexion
C8	Thumb extension
T1	Finger abduction
L1, L2	Hip flexion
L3	Knee extension
L4	Ankle dorsiflexion
L5	Big toe extension
S1	Ankle plantarflexion
S2	Knee flexion

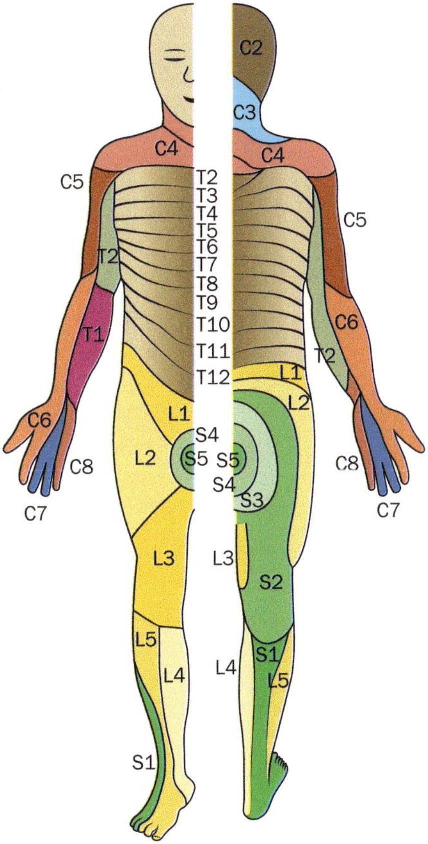

Figure 3.2 Dermatomes and myotomes.

Table 3.3 Special tests for specific conditions.

Test	Condition	Positive finding
Spurling's test – only perform if not irritable; compression of cervical spine in flexion rotation (Figure 3.3)	Radiculopathy	Pain radiates down arm (Childs et al., 2008)
Hoffman's/Tromner sign – flick middle fingertip to see if the thumb and index finger flex involuntarily; positive test indicates myelopathy	Myelopathy	Hyper-reflexia (Nouri et al., 2015)

(Continued)

Table 3.3 (*Continued*)

Test	Condition	Positive finding
Lhermitte's sign – cervical spine flexion in supine with arms and legs flat by the side of body (Figure 3.4)	Spinal cord compression/ multiple sclerosis	Electric shock-like sensation (Thomas et al., 2019)
Romberg's test – checking balance with 30 seconds eyes open then closed to see if patient sways (Figure 3.5)	Ataxia/balance impairment	Balance impairment (Bogduk, 2012)

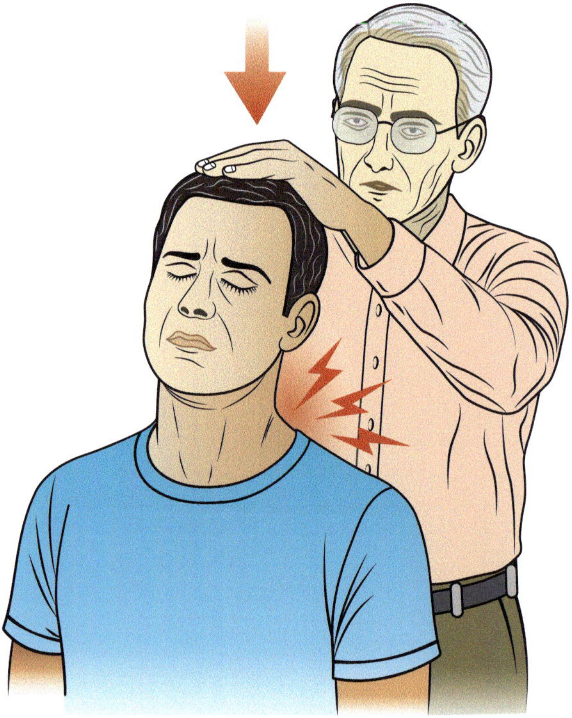

Figure 3.3 Spurling test for cervical radiculopathy. Neck is tilted towards the affected side. Downward pressure is applied to the top of the head to reproduce symptoms of cervical radiculopathy.

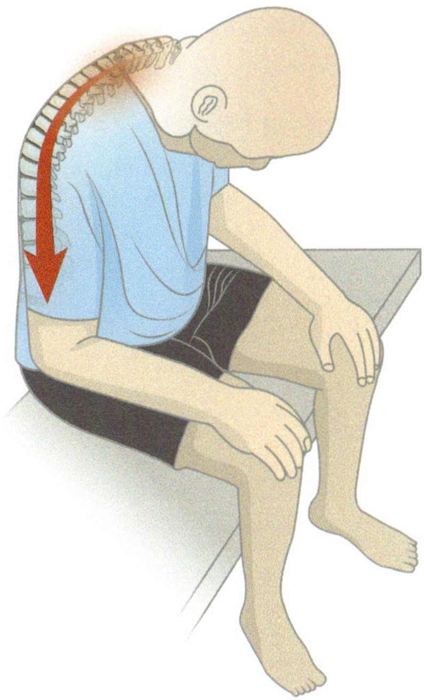

Figure 3.4 Lhermitte's sign. Lhermitte's sign is a sudden sensation that feels like an electric shock running from the neck down the spine, sometimes radiating out to the limbs and extremities.

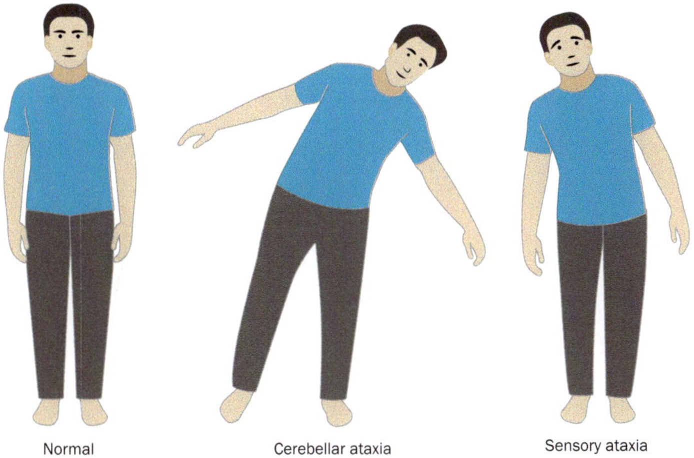

Figure 3.5 Romberg's test.

Management Strategies for Cervical Spine Conditions

Conservative Management in Primary Care

- **Holistic approach:** Suggest ergonomic adjustments, activity modification, reassurance, functional rehabilitation, offer psychological support or signpost to relevant local mental health support team.
- **Physiotherapy:** Refer to physiotherapy for mobility and strengthening treatments.
- **Pain relief:** Prescribe NSAIDs if tolerated, suggest over-the-counter paracetamol, or prescribe muscle relaxants
- **Referral to pain management team:** for chronic persisting neck pain symptoms (Gross et al., 2016).

Interventional Management (When Conservative Treatment Fails)

- **Corticosteroid injections:** For radicular pain, refer to spinal team (Jensen et al., 2022).
- **Surgical referral:** For severe symptoms and pain management.
  - For cervical stenosis with progressive symptoms.
  - For cervical myelopathy.
  - For severe, unremitting radiculopathy (Nouri et al., 2015).

Key Takeaways

Assessment and Differentiation of Mechanical Neck Pain and Headaches

Distinguishing mechanical neck pain and associated headaches from more serious underlying pathology is crucial in clinical practice. Clinicians should maintain a high index of suspicion and systematically evaluate each patient to ensure that potentially life-threatening conditions are not missed.

Assessment for Neurological and Vascular Red Flags

It is essential always to assess for the presence of neurological symptoms and vascular red flags. Key vascular indicators include the '5 Ds' (dizziness, diplopia, dysarthria, dysphagia, drop attacks) and the '3 Ns' (nausea, nystagmus, numbness). The identification of any of these red flags should prompt consideration of more serious pathology.

Structured Clinical Approach

A structured approach should be adopted, incorporating a thorough history, a comprehensive physical examination and appropriate utilisation of special tests, as outlined by Childs et al. (2008). This systematic process aids in both the identification and exclusion of serious conditions.

Urgent Referral and Investigations

Urgent referral is warranted in the presence of signs suggesting cord compression or infection. If cord compression is suspected, immediate onward referral is essential. For patients presenting with neurological deficits, an MRI scan is the investigation of choice. In cases of trauma, X-ray or CT imaging should be considered the gold standard, in accordance with the recommendations from NICE (2023c).

Table 3.4 Cervical spine clinical scenarios: pattern recognition and red flags.

Clinical scenario	Key clinical tests/ observations	Likely diagnosis/ pattern	Red flags/additional considerations
1. 30-year-old female with migraine history, neck pain, jaw pain, stress-related headaches; onset is chronic, sedentary worker	• Cervical muscle tightness and jaw dysfunction • Clenching/ bruxism • Headache linked to stress and posture at work	Cervicogenic headache with temporomandibular dysfunction (TMD)	Conservative management – refer to physiotherapy • Biopsychosocial contributors • Address sleep, stress, ergonomics The absence of red flags and the presence of consistent mechanical features supported a conservative management approach, with clear safety netting provided

(Continued)

Table 3.4 *(Continued)*

Clinical scenario	Key clinical tests/ observations	Likely diagnosis/ pattern	Red flags/additional considerations
2. 46-year-old female supermarket worker with neck pain, right arm numbness and weakness, worse with dressing, onset is acute	• Dermatomal sensory loss • Reduced myotome strength • Pain increased with cervical extension	Cervical radiculopathy	Conservative management – refer to physiotherapy • Consider MRI if persistent or progressive – refer to secondary care • Monitor neurological deficit • Escalate referral to neurology if worsening The absence of red flags and the presence of consistent mechanical features supported a conservative management approach, with clear safety netting provided
3. 67-year-old female with neck stiffness, bilateral pins and needles, foot catching, imbalance, angina history, onset of new symptoms is acute	• Hyper-reflexia • Ataxic gait • Positive Hoffmann's/ Babinski • Symptoms worsen with cervical extension	Degenerative cervical myelopathy ± cervical arterial dysfunction – considering cardiovascular history	Urgent referral to spine service for ⚐ Urgent MRI ⚐ Possible spinal cord compression ⚐ Vascular risk – urgent referral required

Clinical scenario	Key clinical tests/ observations	Likely diagnosis/ pattern	Red flags/additional considerations
4. 22-year-old female student post bike accident with neck pain, headaches, blurred vision, arm pain, poor sleep, anxiety, onset is acute	• Neck pain and stiffness • Sensorimotor control deficits • Psychological distress	Whiplash-associated disorder (WAD) – Grade II/III	Conservative management – refer to physiotherapy Screen for post-traumatic disorder The absence of red flags and the presence of consistent mechanical features supported a conservative management approach, with clear safety netting provided
5. 38-year-old male sedentary desk worker with neck and hand symptoms, right fingers are tingling, right hand is fatigued, worse with typing, onset is 2 months	• Positive Spurling's test • Positive Phalen's or Tinel's – for carpal tunnel syndrome • Reduced grip strength • Incomplete symptom resolution with neck physiotherapy	Double crush syndrome (cervical radiculopathy + carpal tunnel syndrome)	Conservative management – refer to physiotherapy. The absence of red flags and the presence of consistent mechanical features supported a conservative management approach, with clear safety netting provided Dual-site nerve compression: • Requires cervical and peripheral assessment • Treat both sites concurrently

CHAPTER 4

The Thoracic Spine

Introduction

The thoracic spine is recognised as the least mobile yet most stable section of the vertebral column. This stability is largely attributed to its firm attachment to the ribcage. The thoracic spine serves several crucial functions, including providing postural support, facilitating respiration, supporting the thoracic viscera and contributing significantly to the overall stability of the spine (Standring, 2021). A substantial proportion of adults, about 30–50%, report thoracic pain, which can result in recurrent pain and stiffness, with symptoms that may be felt not only in the thoracic area but also referred to the chest, upper back or even the arms and legs (Bogduk, 2012). Thoracic pain is more prevalent in females and commonly seen in sedentary workers, affecting functional limitation and leading to sleep disturbances and reduced working ability (Cagnie et al., 2013).

Anatomy of the Thoracic Spine

The thoracic spine is composed of twelve vertebrae, designated T1 to T12, each of which articulates with the ribs and sternum (Figure 4.1). Several key anatomical structures are essential to its function.

- **Vertebral bodies**: These structures are responsible for supporting weight-bearing forces throughout the thoracic region.
- **Intervertebral discs**: Positioned between each vertebra, these discs allow for controlled movement and act as shock absorbers.
- **Facet joints**: These joints guide and limit the movement of the thoracic spine, contributing to its stability and mobility.

- **Costovertebral and costotransverse joints**: These joints serve as the connection points between the ribs and the spine, facilitating the mechanics of breathing.
- **Spinal cord and nerve roots**: The thoracic spine houses and protects the spinal cord and nerve roots, which are vital for controlling sensory and motor function in the trunk and lower limbs (Standring, 2021).

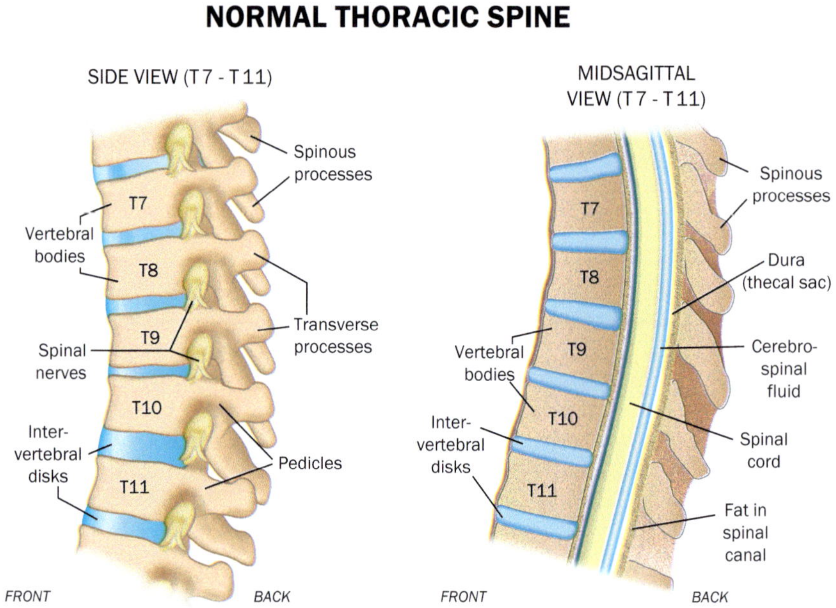

Figure 4.1 Thoracic spine anatomical structures.

Common Thoracic Spine Conditions and Red Flags

Table 4.1 details the most common thoracic spine conditions seen in primary care, while Table 4.2 presents the red flags to be aware of in thoracic spine disorders. Thoracic pain is **less commonly mechanical** than cervical or lumbar pain and should prompt careful consideration of serious pathology (Bogduk, 2012). Common Thoracic conditions seen in primary care are listed in (Table 4.3).

Table 4.1 Common thoracic spine conditions.

Condition	Cause	Symptoms	Investigations	Management
Mechanical thoracic pain	Poor posture, muscle strain, joint dysfunction Any age	Localised mid-back pain, stiffness	Clinical diagnosis with palpation of thoracic spine and neurological examination, X-ray if persistent after 6 weeks	Refer to physiotherapy, ergonomic changes, NSAIDs* (Briggs et al., 2021)
Thoracic disc herniation	Trauma, degenerative changes Middle age onwards	Radicular pain, myelopathy, sensory deficits	MRI (gold standard) via secondary care referral	Refer to physiotherapy, NSAIDs*, surgical decompression if severe (Court et al., 2017)
Scheuermann's kyphosis	Adolescent vertebral growth abnormalities <16 years old	Postural kyphosis, back pain	Confirm with X-ray (Schmorl's nodes)	Refer to physiotherapy Postural correction, bracing, Pilates physiotherapy, surgery only required if severe (Bagnall et al., 2008)
Thoracic myelopathy	Spinal cord compression from stenosis, disc herniation, trauma, space-occupying lesions, etc. Any age	Gait disturbances, lower limb weakness, hyper-reflexia	MRI via secondary care referral	Decompression surgery if referral to physiotherapy does not resolve symptoms (Nouri et al., 2015)

(Continued)

Table 4.1 (*Continued*)

Condition	Cause	Symptoms	Investigations	Management
Thoracic outlet syndrome (TOS)	Compression of brachial plexus, subclavian artery or vein Females > males	Arm pain, paraesthesia, swelling (vascular cases), weak grip, cold hand	Clinical tests (Adson's, Roos), Doppler ultrasound, MR angiography for vascular cases via secondary care referral	Refer to physiotherapy (first line for neurogenic TOS), botulinum toxin injections, surgical decompression for vascular cases (Hooper et al., 2010; Illig et al., 2016)

*NSAIDs – if allowed and tolerated or start with paracetamol.

Abbreviations: MR, magnetic resonancc; NSAID, non-steroidal anti-inflammatory drug.

Table 4.2 Red flags in thoracic spine disorders.

Red flag symptoms	Potential serious condition	Immediate action
Severe unremitting pain, night pain that does not resolve with rest or movement, loss of appetite, unexplained weight loss >5 % of body weight in the past 6–12 months, fever/chills, malaise, fatigue	Malignancy, infection	Gold standard – MRI, two-week cancer referral (Nouri et al., 2015)
Bilateral sensory loss, upper limb weakness, hyper-reflexia	Thoracic myelopathy	Urgent MRI via secondary care referral, followed by neurosurgery referral (Court et al., 2017)
New-onset thoracic pain with fever, unexplained weight loss, malaise, fatigue	Spinal infection (discitis, osteomyelitis)	Urgent blood tests (CRP, ESR), MRI via emergency referral and antibiotics (Briggs et al., 2021)
Acute chest pain with back pain radiation	Aortic dissection, pulmonary embolism	Emergency referral for imaging (Illig et al., 2016)

Abbreviations: CRP, C-reactive protein; ESR, erythrocyte sedimentation rate; MRI, magnetic resonance imaging.

Diagnostic Approach for Thoracic Spine Disorders

Clinical Examination

- **Inspection:** Posture deviations – kyphosis, scoliosis, muscle atrophy, anatomical deviations, swelling/lumps/bumps, skin colour changes.
- **Palpation:** Tenderness, muscle tightness, rib dysfunction.
- **Range of motion (ROM):** Flexion, extension, rotation, side bending.
- **Neurological testing**: Reflexes (Figure 4.2), dermatomes (T1–T12) (see Figure 3.2), myotomes (Court et al., 2017).

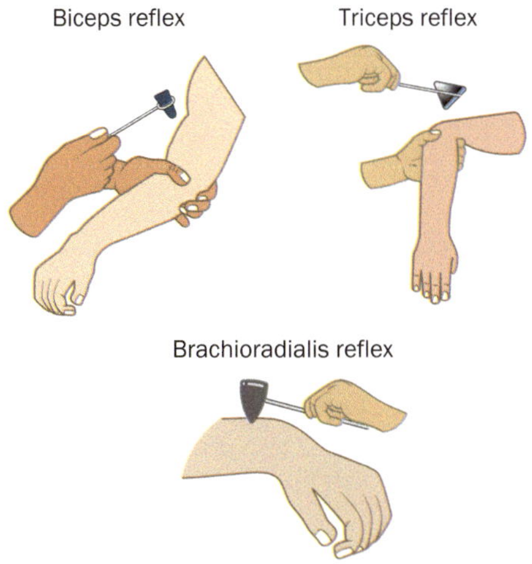

Figure 4.2 Reflex testing in cervical and thoracic spine.

Imaging and Investigations

- X-ray (first line of investigation for fractures, scoliosis).
- Refer for MRI via secondary care (gold standard for soft tissue pathology, myelopathy, disc herniation) (Nouri et al., 2015).
- CT scan via secondary care (best for bony abnormalities, surgical planning) (Briggs et al., 2021).
- Blood tests – for spine infection and malignancies; can be done in primary care (Briggs et al., 2021).

Key Takeaways

Conditions affecting the thoracic spine frequently arise from issues related to posture or mechanical dysfunction, or may be indicative of more serious underlying pathology. It is important to distinguish between these origins to ensure appropriate management and referral pathways.

Thoracic Outlet Syndrome

Thoracic outlet syndrome is a commonly misdiagnosed condition that involves neurovascular structures. Accurate diagnosis of this syndrome necessitates a thorough clinical examination combined with appropriate imaging techniques, as highlighted by Illig et al. (2016).

Recognition of Serious Pathology

Serious red flag presentations, such as neurological deficits, persistent or unremitting pain and the presence of systemic symptoms, must be identified quickly. These findings should prompt urgent referral to a specialist for further evaluation, as advised by Bogduk (2012).

Role of Imaging

Magnetic resonance imaging is the gold standard for assessing spinal cord compression and disc pathology. Referral to secondary care for MRI is warranted when such conditions are suspected, in accordance with the recommendations of Court et al. (2017).

Visceral Causes of Thoracic Pain

It should be noted that thoracic pain may sometimes be related to viscera (heart, spleen, liver, gall bladder, pancreas, stomach, kidney) but mimic MSK symptoms. Therefore, a comprehensive patient history and thorough clinical examination are essential for accurate diagnosis and management.

Table 4.3 Thoracic spine clinical scenarios: pattern recognition and red flags.

Clinical scenario	Key clinical tests/ observations	Likely diagnosis/ pattern	Red flags/ additional considerations
1. 22-year-old female, family history of rheumatoid arthritis, dull chest pain + thoracic pain, rib cage is tender, cardiac causes are ruled out, chronic onset of pain	Decreased thoracic expansion Costovertebral tenderness Inflammatory pattern (morning stiffness, early morning waking, pain with rest, better with movement)	Inflammatory axial (spondyloarthropathy)	Urgent rheumatology referral MRI whole spine recommended Physiotherapy referral for rehabilitation

Clinical scenario	Key clinical tests/ observations	Likely diagnosis/ pattern	Red flags/ additional considerations
2. 78-year-old female, acute thoracic pain after changing bed sheets; known osteopenia, hypertension, history of smoking – 4/day, lives alone, independent, keep fit class 1/ week	Spinal tenderness on percussion (percuss on spinous process where the pain is reported) Painful standing for >10 min	Vertebral compression fracture	X-ray – first line of investigations MRI – secondary care referral Screen for sinister pathologies
3. 52-year-old male, history of bowel cancer (10 years ago), thoracic back pain with sleep, reduced mobility and function	Pain not relieved by rest Night pain that disturbs sleep Prior cancer history	Spinal metastasis	MRI spine required via urgent suspected cancer pathway referral if unexplained weight loss + systemic signs
4. 34-year-old male, fit and active gym instructor, reported acute arm heaviness/ numbness, thoracic pains worsened with overhead activity	Positive Roos or Adson's test Increased symptoms with arm elevation Not following a specific dermatomal pattern Vascular assessment	Thoracic outlet syndrome (TOS)	Refer to physiotherapy and imaging is required to discern if neurogenic or vascular in nature Refer to vascular team if pulses are affected
5. 42-year-old obese female, desk worker, reported mid-thoracic pain, onset of 2 months, large breasts, otherwise well systemically	Pain worse after sitting No red flags reported for cancer or infection Relieved by movement/postural correction	Mechanical thoracic pain	Education about movement + ergonomics Refer to physiotherapy for thoracic mobility + scapular control + support

CHAPTER 5

The Lumbar Spine

Introduction

Low back pain (LBP) is the most prevalent musculoskeletal condition globally and remains the leading cause of years lived with disability (YLDs) according to the most recent Global Burden of Disease analysis (GBD 2021 Low Back Pain Collaborators, 2023). Lifetime prevalence estimates suggest that up to 80% of adults will experience LBP at some point in their lives, with annual prevalence rates of 30–40% consistently reported across population studies (NHS Digital, 2022; NICE, 2020).

In the UK, approximately one in six adults reports back pain at any given time, and around 20% live with chronic LBP persisting for more than three months (NHS Digital, 2022). LBP has substantial socio-economic impact, accounting for around 12–13% of lost working days and contributing to nearly 30% of all UK sickness absence (ONS, 2023).

The financial cost is considerable, with estimates suggesting that low back pain costs the UK economy £10–12.3 billion annually, including healthcare expenditure and productivity losses, while the NHS alone spends over £2.1 billion each year managing back pain in primary and secondary care (NHS England, 2021; NICE, 2020).

Recurrence is also common, with 60–70% of individuals experiencing a new episode within a year, and approximately 20% of acute cases progressing to chronicity (NICE, 2020). Together, these findings highlight the pervasive clinical, social and economic burden of lumbar spine pain across the UK and internationally.

Problems that affect the lumbar spine are among the most prevalent sources of musculoskeletal pain. Such conditions can lead to considerable levels of disability in addition to financial burden across the globe, impacting daily activities and quality of life (NICE, 2023a). Common conditions are listed in Table 5.1 and red flags for lumbar spine are listed in Table 5.2.

Table 5.1 Common lumbar spine conditions.

Condition	Cause	Symptoms	Investigations	Management
Mechanical low back pain/non-specific low back pain	Multifaceted causes, muscle strain, overuse, underuse, psychosocial, insidious onset	Localised pain, stiffness, occasional psychosomatic referral patterns Age – varied	Clinical diagnosis utilising subjective and objective examination	Referral to physiotherapy, NSAIDs*, ergonomic changes, functional rehabilitation and psychological support (Foster et al., 2018)
Lumbar disc herniation	Degenerative disc disease, trauma/injury, insidious onset Sudden movements	Localised pain, radicular pain, weakness in leg muscles, paraesthesia – sensory deficits Age – varied	Referral to secondary care for MRI (gold standard) only if symptoms do not resolve with conservative management	Conservative management – referral to physiotherapy, psychological support, prescribe NSAIDs*, surgical decompression if severe – via neurosurgery/spine team referral (Jensen et al., 2022)

Lumbar canal stenosis	Degenerative alterations, osteophyte formation, insufficient or excessive joint use, obesity, Insidious	Neurogenic claudication, bilateral leg weakness and pains. Mostly >50 years old Low back and leg pains with standing and walking Classic trolley sign – patient wants to lean forward to relieve pains Sitting is easier than standing or walking	Referral to secondary care for MRI if symptoms do not resolve with conservative management	Conservative management – referral to physiotherapy, exercises, activity modification, surgery if severe – via neurosurgery/spine team referral (Nouri et al., 2015)
Spondylolisthesis	Vertebral slippage due to fracture or degeneration	Low back pain, leg symptoms, referred symptoms, motor weakness in legs, sensory deficits Young as well as older patient population	Primary care investigation – X-ray, MRI if neurological symptoms via secondary care referral	Physiotherapy referral, activity modification, core strengthening, surgery if unstable spine via referral to spine/neurosurgery team (Kalichman et al., 2009)

*NSAIDs – if allowed/tolerated or start with paracetamol.

Abbreviations: MRI, magnetic resonance imaging; NSAID, non-steroidal anti-inflammatory drug.

Table 5.2 Lumbar spine red flags and referral criteria - screening for serious pathology (NICE 2023a).

Red flag	Potential serious condition	Immediate action
Progressive back pain not relieved by rest, unremitting night pain, unexplained weight loss >5% of body weight in the past 6–12 months, fever, malaise, fatigue, leg weakness and decreased function/movement	Malignancy, infection	MRI via urgent suspected cancer pathway (Finucane et al., 2020; Nouri et al., 2015)
Overflow bladder incontinence, flaccid anus, sexual dysfunction, saddle anaesthesia, bilateral paraesthesia	Cauda equina syndrome	Urgent emergency, neurosurgery referral (GIRFT, 2023; Goubran and Tomlinson, 2023)
Recent infection, fever/chills, spinal tenderness, fatigue	Spinal infection (discitis, osteomyelitis)	Urgent blood tests (CRP, ESR), MRI via secondary care referral (Briggs et al., 2021; Salisbury et al., 2022a).
Severe back pain, fatigue, tiredness, anaemia, hypercalcaemia, pain unchanged with position and spinal tenderness	Multiple myeloma	MRI via secondary care referral/emergency referral, urgent two-week referral (Stewart, 2005)

Abbreviations: CRP, C-reactive protein; ESR, erythrocyte sedimentation rate; MRI, magnetic resonance imaging.

Anatomy of the Lumbar Spine

The lumbar spine is composed of five vertebrae, labelled L1 to L5. These vertebrae are responsible for striking a balance between stability and mobility within the lower back region. The structural elements of the lumbar spine each play a distinct role in its overall function (Figure 5.1).

- **Vertebral bodies:** These are the principal load-bearing structures, supporting the weight of the upper body.
- **Intervertebral disc**s: Located between the vertebrae, these discs act as shock absorbers and facilitate movement by allowing flexibility and stability.
- **Facet joints:** These joints help control the degree and direction of movement within the spine, contributing to its mobility.

- **Nerve roots (L1–S1):** Emerging from the lumbar spine, these nerve roots provide innervation to the lower limbs, playing a crucial role in motor and sensory function (Bogduk, 2012).

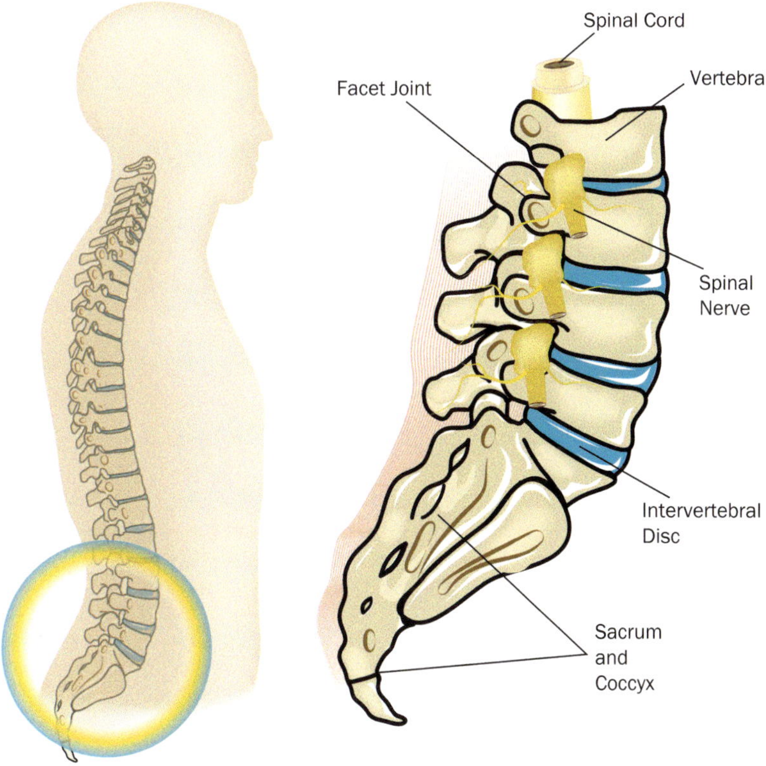

Figure 5.1 Lumbar spine anatomical structures.

Diagnostic Approach for Lumbar Spine Disorders

Clinical Examination

- **Observation** – Posture, gait, spinal curvature, anatomical deviations.
- **Palpation** – Tenderness, muscle spasm, muscle tightness.
- **Range of motion (ROM)** – Flexion, extension, side flexion, rotation.
- **Neurological testing** – Reflexes (Figure 5.2), dermatomes (L1–S2, see Figure 3.2), myotomes (Figure 5.3), Babinski (Figure 5.4), clonus test (Figure 5.5), gait, balance, co-ordination and functional tests, heel–toe walk, single-leg and double-leg squat (Court et al., 2017).

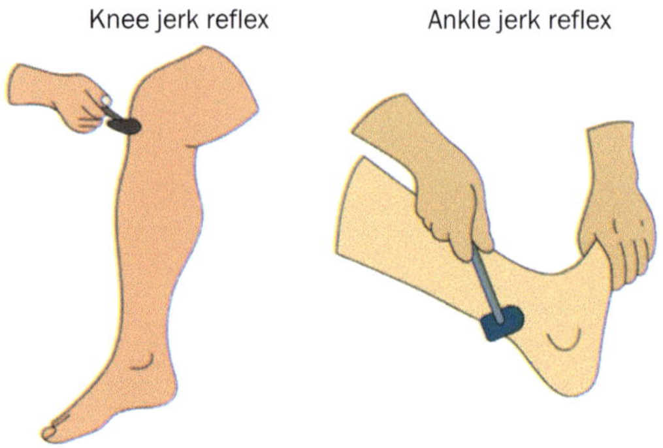

Figure 5.2 Lower limb reflexes.

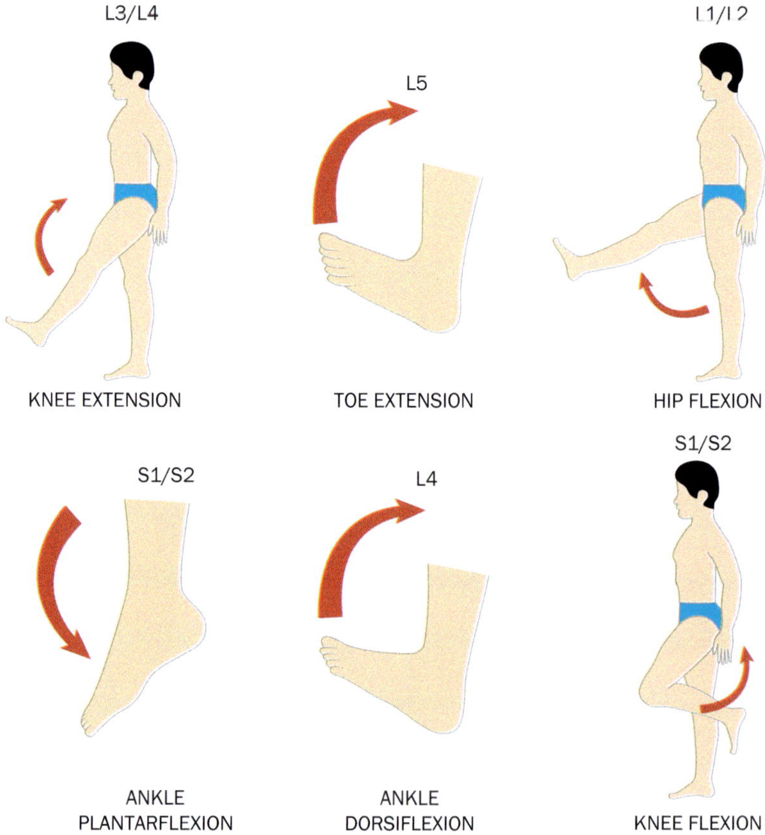

Figure 5.3 Myotomes.

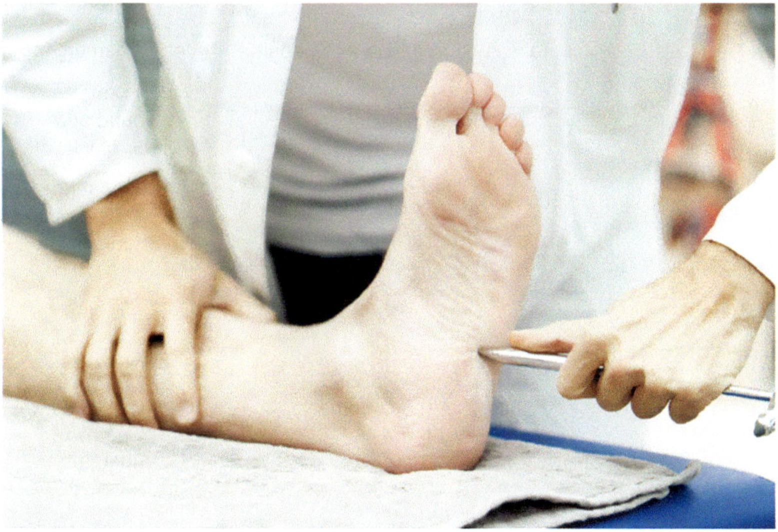

Figure 5.4 Babinski sign. Down-going plantars – normal. Up-going plantars indicate neurological dysfunction.

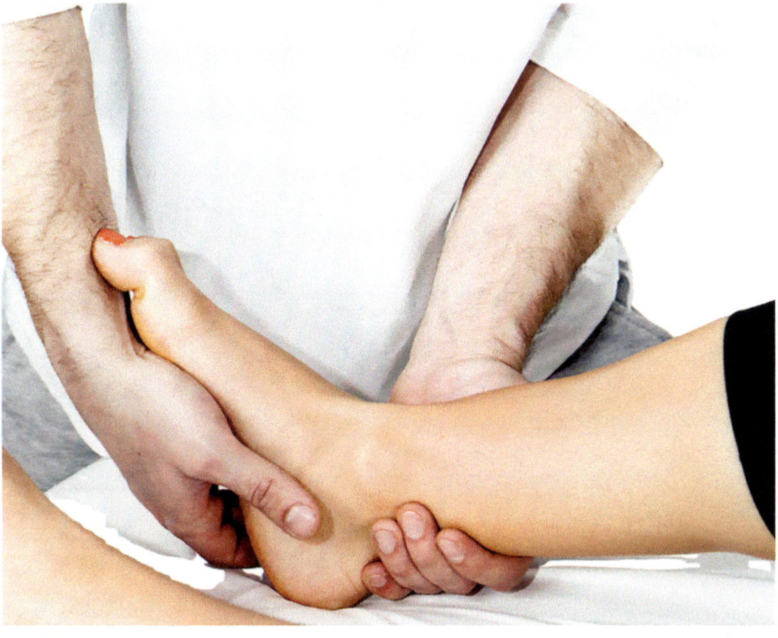

Figure 5.5 Clonus test. >3 involuntary beats with ankle dorsiflexion indicates neurological dysfunction.

Imaging and Investigations

- **X-ray** – First line of investigation for trauma/fractures, spondylolisthesis.
- **MRI** – Gold standard for disc herniation, stenosis, malignancy via secondary care referrals (Nouri et al., 2015).
- **CT scan** – Best for bony abnormalities via secondary care referrals (Briggs et al., 2021).

Management Strategies for Lumbar Spine Conditions

Conservative Management

- **Refer to physiotherapy** – Core strengthening, mobility exercises and reassurance.
- **Pain relief** – Suggest over-the-counter NSAIDs or paracetamol, prescribe stronger NSAIDS such as naproxen if age >65 then proton pump inhibitors (PPI) such as omeprazole/lansoprazole (Foster et al., 2018).
- **Lifestyle modifications** – Suggest microbreaks for sedentary workforce and ergonomic interventions.
- **Psychology** – Suggest talking therapies and mindfulness practices; provide education.

Interventional Management (When Conservative Treatment Fails)

- **Epidural steroid injections** – For radicular pain (Jensen et al., 2022) via secondary care referrals to pain management.
- **Surgical referral:**
  - For lumbar stenosis with progressive symptoms.
  - For lumbar disc herniation causing severe radiculopathy (Nouri et al., 2015).

Key Takeaways

Non-surgical Management of Low Back Pain

The management of low back pain frequently involves a combination of physiotherapy, psychological support and the encouragement of regular walking and movement. These approaches have been shown to enhance recovery and contribute to improved patient outcomes, illustrated in the low back pain pathway in (Figure 5.6).

Physiotherapy

Engaging in physiotherapy enables patients to strengthen their core muscles, improve flexibility and regain function, which in turn helps to alleviate discomfort and restore mobility.

PATIENT WITH LOW BACK PAIN (+/- LEG PAIN)

(NICE NG59 [NICE, 2016a] Low Back Pain ± Sciatica Pathway)

Take history and examination:
- Mechanism, duration
- Neuro screen
- Red flags (cancer, infection, fracture, CE)?

RED FLAGS PRESENT?

YES

Emergency/urgent medical pathway (as appropriate)

NO

Classify pain:
- Non-specific LBP
- LBP with sciatica

FIRST-LINE MANAGEMENT (NO RED FLAGS):
- Reassure, explain benign nature (in majority)
- Encourage activity and early return to work
- Structured exercise programme
- Consider manual therapy ONLY as part of package with exercise
- Screen psychosocial factors (yellow flags)

REVIEW AFTER A PERIOD (e.g. 4–6 WEEKS)

IMPROVING/STABLE

Optimise conservative management; Continue self-management; Progress exercises.

NOT IMPROVING OR WORSE

Consider step-down review; MRI/specialist opinion/(radiculopathy); Severe neurological deficit; Reassess diagnosis and red flags; Consider neuropathic features; Consider surgery or invasive procedure.

Figure 5.6 Low back pain pathway.

Psychological Support

Psychological support is an essential component of care, as it addresses the emotional and mental impact of chronic pain. Supporting patients in managing stress and anxiety can foster resilience and promote a more positive outlook during recovery.

Walking and Movement

Regular walking and movement is vital for maintaining activity levels and preventing deconditioning. Gradual increases in physical activity can aid in reducing pain and improving overall well-being.

Differentiating and Managing Low Back Pain

Mechanical low back pain should be distinguished from more serious underlying pathologies. It is important to recognise that low back pain is multifaceted and therefore requires a holistic approach to management.

A thorough assessment is essential, paying particular attention to the presence of neurological symptoms and red flags that may indicate more serious conditions (Table 5.3). For example, symptoms suggestive of myeloma or malignancy require further investigation, with referral for MRI via secondary care being the key imaging modality recommended by NICE (2023a).

Clinicians should be vigilant for signs of cauda equina syndrome or infection, as these require urgent referral to secondary care services for immediate assessment and intervention. Patients should be safety netted and documentation of this advice is essential for medicolegal purposes.

Most low back pain patients can be effectively managed through a combination of physiotherapy, psychological support and encouragement of walking and regular movement, all of which contribute to improved outcomes and recovery.

Table 5.3 Lumbar spine clinical scenarios: pattern recognition and red flags.

Clinical scenario	Key clinical tests/ observations	Likely diagnosis/pattern	Red flags/additional considerations
25-year-old male, gym user, reported bilateral leg paraesthesia, groin numbness after a heavy leg day. He reported dead leg 4 days post injury	Saddle anaesthesia Bilateral leg symptoms Reflex changes Increased urinary frequency	Suspected cauda equina syndrome (CES)	This is a surgical emergency and warrants urgent MRI via emergency referral. Immediate neurosurgery referral if cauda equina suspected by emergency doctor
60-year-old male, smoker, past medical history of angina, reported chronic low back + acute-onset abdominal pain and pain radiating to the right thigh	Pulsatile abdominal mass on examination Low blood pressure Sweating	Abdominal aortic aneurysm (AAA) suspected	This is a vascular emergency if rupture is suspected Abdominal ultrasound initially to check the size of aorta and refer to emergency for severe cases
55-year-old female retail worker reported pain with walking 10 min, better with sitting/leaning, grocery shopping aggravates her pain. Bilateral aching in the legs, no weakness, no bladder or bowel symptoms reported	Worse with extension movement Relief with flexion movement Negative straight leg test Neurogenic claudication – symptoms in legs; nerve compression	Lumbar spinal stenosis	MRI spine if worsening symptoms via secondary care referral Flexion-based exercises to aid rehabilitation Refer to physiotherapy Surgical intervention if severe via neurosurgery referral

(*Continued*)

Table 5.3 *(Continued)*

Clinical scenario	Key clinical tests/ observations	Likely diagnosis/pattern	Red flags/additional considerations
48-year-old female runner, reported right lateral hip pain + right-sided back pain, pain is worse lying on side. She is struggling to continue her desk work and running activities	Tenderness over right greater trochanter Single-leg squat is painful on right side Normal lumbar ROM, mild pains on right-sided lumbar flexion	Greater trochanteric pain syndrome (GTPS) can present as lower back pain. It is important to understand the source of symptoms	Physiotherapy referral for hip tendon exercises: progressive loading programme is suggested Avoid side sleeping and cross sitting on right side Also avoid stretches for hip Exercises, topical anti-inflammatory and ice can help
63-year-old male, smoker, reported three months of constant back pain, no relief with medication/movements, recent chest infection, systemic malaise, feeling unwell	Non-mechanical, persistent pain Constant unremitting night pain ↑ Calcium on bone profile Anaemia Bone lesion suspected	Multiple myeloma	Red flags that increase suspicion – age, smoker, systemic signs Urgent MRI spine via emergency referral Bloods: FBC, bone profile, U/E, serum immunoglobulins, urine Bence Jones proteins Refer onwards

Abbreviations: FBC, full blood count; MRI, magnetic resonance imaging; ROM, range of motion; U/E, urea and electrolytes.

CHAPTER 6

The Shoulder

Introduction

Prevalence and Impact of Shoulder Pain

Shoulder pain is a prevalent musculoskeletal complaint encountered in primary care settings. The point prevalence of shoulder pain in the general adult population ranges between 15% and 30%, while annual prevalence estimates vary from 20% to 50%, influenced by demographic factors (Luime et al., 2004). Notably, the lifetime prevalence of shoulder pain may reach up to 70%, highlighting the considerable burden of shoulder dysfunction throughout the lifespan (Mitchell et al., 2005).

Within UK primary care, shoulder pain accounts for approximately 14% of all musculoskeletal complaints. It is the third most common reason for a musculoskeletal consultation, surpassed only by low back and knee pain (Mitchell et al., 2005). Chronic shoulder pain is a frequent issue, with research indicating that 40–50% of affected individuals continue to experience symptoms after twelve months. Furthermore, up to 25% of those affected may develop persistent limitations in their daily functional abilities (Van der Windt et al., 2010).

Demographics and Functional Consequences

Shoulder pain is most frequently observed between the ages of 45 and 65, a tendency that reflects degenerative changes in the rotator cuff associated with ageing (Luime et al., 2004). The impact of shoulder pain extends beyond physical discomfort, as it significantly affects work capacity, leading to work disability, reduced productivity and extended periods of sickness absence.

Consequently, shoulder pain constitutes a major contributor to the overall musculoskeletal burden, particularly among the working-age population.

Underlying Causes and Joint Vulnerability

The shoulder is among the most mobile joints in the human body, allowing for a wide range of movements. However, this mobility can compromise the joint's stability, rendering it more susceptible to injuries and various dysfunctions (Standring, 2021). In primary care, shoulder conditions frequently arise due to traumatic incidents, repetitive overuse, degenerative changes associated with ageing or ongoing instability of the joint. Each of these factors plays a role in the development and persistence of shoulder pathology (Lewis et al., 2015). Some of the common shoulder conditions are listed in Table 6.1 and red flags to be vigilant for are listed in Table 6.2.

Anatomy of the Shoulder

The shoulder complex consists of the following aspects (Figure 6.1).

- **Glenohumeral joint (GHJ)** – Ball-and-socket joint between head of humerus and scapular glenoid cavity providing mobility.
- **Acromioclavicular joint (ACJ)** – Joint between acromion and clavicle which supports load transfer from the upper limb.
- **Sternoclavicular joint (SCJ)** – Joint between sternum and clavicle which connects the shoulder to the axial skeleton.
- **Scapulothoracic articulation** – Allows smooth shoulder motion (Standring 2021).

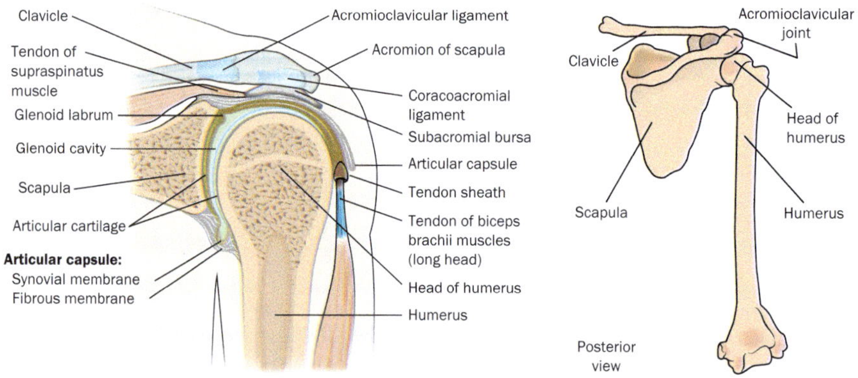

Figure 6.1 Shoulder anatomy.

Table 6.1 Common shoulder conditions.

Condition	Cause	Symptoms	Investigations	Management
Rotator cuff-related pain syndrome (RCRPS)	Overuse, degeneration, insidious onset Inflammatory condition – axial spondyloarthropathy	Painful shoulder abduction and rotation at 90° and overhead Weakness in arm muscles	Referral for ultrasound via secondary care, if no improvement then MRI if not improving with conservative management and injection	Physiotherapy referral and NSAIDs*, corticosteroid injections if pain and lack of function are impairing quality of life (Lewis, 2016)
Rotator cuff tear	Trauma, degenerative changes Any age	Weakness in the arm, night pain, difficulty lifting arm overhead, dressing and undressing issues affecting quality of life	MRI (gold standard) via secondary referral if symptoms worsened	Physiotherapy referral and surgical repair if full-thickness tear is debilitating the function in some cases (Diercks et al., 2014)
Frozen shoulder (adhesive capsulitis)	Idiopathic, post-injury, diabetes related, thyroid related, hypertension can trigger, hormonal changes, metabolic factors, age 40–60 Females > Males	Progressive stiffness, pain related to shoulder movements – flexion, abduction, hand behind back and hand behind head	Clinical diagnosis using capsular pattern of shoulder. Limited shoulder flexion, abduction and external rotation. Limited external rotation is clinical sign to confirm frozen shoulder. X-ray to rule out joint conditions if suspected but not mandatory. Three phases – painful phase, stiffness phase and resolution phase	Resolution of symptoms in 2–4 years. Physiotherapy referral NSAIDs*, intra-articular steroid injection in the initial phase (Wang et al., 2017)

(*Continued*)

Table 6.1 *(Continued)*

Condition	Cause	Symptoms	Investigations	Management
Shoulder instability (dislocation)	Trauma, congenital laxity in shoulder ligaments, hypermobility syndrome conditions Any age	Recurrent dislocations, shoulder pain, 90° shoulder abduction and external rotation – painful	X-ray (to rule out fracture initially), MRI for soft tissue assessment to rule out tears via secondary referral	Physiotherapy referral for conservative management and surgical stabilisation if recurrent (Longo et al., 2011)
Acromioclavicular joint (ACJ) sprain	Direct trauma (fall on shoulder), overuse Any age	ACJ tenderness, swelling, pain with overhead movement, difficulty in daily activities	X-ray (graded Rockwood classification) to determine the extent of injury which in turn dictates the prognosis	NSAIDs* – topical/over the counter/prescribed, shoulder sling via fracture clinic referral, physiotherapy referral to restore movement and function (Beitzel et al., 2014)
Osteoarthritis (GHJ or ACJ)	Cartilage degeneration limiting movement Age >40	Crepitus, stiffness, deep shoulder pain and restrictions with activities and sleeping	X-ray (joint space narrowing, osteophytes)	NSAIDs*, physiotherapy referral, steroid injections for pain relief and improving quality of life, followed by total shoulder replacement if there are severe restrictions resulting in poor quality of life (Papalia et al., 2020)
Labral tears, SLAP lesions, Hill-Sachs lesions	Shoulder labral disorders due to trauma, sports, overuse, degeneration of shoulder labrum Any age	Pain with elevation, abduction, rotation movements, weakness in arm muscles, painful 90° flexion, painful resisted flexion movement	MRI to confirm the lesion and extent via secondary care referral	Physiotherapy referral for progressive loading rehabilitation programme, surgical repair based on the extent of the tears (Lewis et al., 2015).

*NSAIDs – if allowed or start with paracetamol.

Abbreviations: GHJ, glenohumeral joint; MRI, magnetic resonance imaging; NSAID, non-steroidal anti-inflammatory drug; SLAP, superior labrum anterior to posterior.

Table 6.2 Red flags in shoulder disorders.

Red flag	Potential serious condition	Immediate action
Sudden-onset shoulder pain with fever/chills, systemic illness such as chest infection or urinary tract infection, etc.	Septic arthritis	Urgent referral to emergency joint aspiration, IV antibiotics (Mathews et al., 2010)
Persistent, non-mechanical shoulder pain, unremitting night pain, unexplained weight loss	Malignancy, metastases	Urgent MRI via urgent suspected cancer pathway, oncology referral (Lewis et al., 2015)
Acute pain post trauma with deformity, loss of function	Fracture, dislocation	X-ray as first line of investigation, urgent orthopaedic referral if severe symptoms occur (Beitzel et al., 2014)
Neurological symptoms in the arm (numbness, weakness, wasting of muscles)	Brachial plexus injury, cervical radiculopathy – severe nerve compression	Referral to MRI via secondary care, nerve conduction studies (Papalia et al., 2020)

Abbreviations: IV, intravenous; MRI, magnetic resonance imaging.

Assessment Approach for Shoulder Disorders

Clinical Examination

- **Observation** – Skin colour changes, swelling/inflammation, anatomical variations, muscle wasting, atrophy, winging of scapula (long thoracic nerve palsy).
- **Palpation** – ACJ, rotator cuff insertion, GHJ capsule.
- **Range of motion (ROM)** – Active and passive movement assessment (Standring 2021).
- **Muscle strengthening** – resisted movement to assess muscle strength.

Special Tests

These tests (Table 6.3 and Figure 6.2) help with assessment and diagnosis but are not considered to be reliable or valid. Clinical scenarios and management listed in Table 6.4.

Table 6.3 Special tests for shoulder conditions.

Test	Condition	Positive finding
Neer's test	Rotator cuff-related pain syndrome	Pain with internally rotated arm in elevation (Lewis, 2016)
Hawkins–Kennedy test	Rotator cuff-related pain syndrome	Pain at 90° abduction + elbow flexion and internal rotation (Diercks et al., 2014)
Apprehension test	Shoulder instability	Feeling of instability, pain with shoulder in 90° abduction and external rotation (Longo et al., 2011)
Speed's test	Biceps tendinopathy	Pain over bicipital groove with resisted shoulder flexion in elbow extension (Beitzel et al., 2014)
External rotation test	Frozen shoulder	Pain and stiffness in active as well as passive external rotation of shoulder (Brady et al., 2020)
Painful arc test	Rotator cuff-related pain syndrome	Painful shoulder abduction over 90°, extended elbow position (Yazigi, 2021)
Drop arm test	Rotator cuff tear test	Weakness in lifting the arm overhead (Yazigi, 2021; Littlewood et al., 2020)

Table 6.4 Clinical scenarios for shoulder conditions.

Clinical scenarios	Symptoms/conditions	Diagnosis	Causes
45-year-old female, desk worker, insidious onset of shoulder pain for two months, struggles to sleep on affected side, no weakness, raised Hb1Ac	Limited external rotation (active and passive): → frozen shoulder	Frozen shoulder (adhesive capsulitis)	Type II diabetes linked with tendon pathology
	Resisted external rotation painful with good ROM: → Rotator cuff-related pain syndrome	Rotator cuff-related pain syndrome	Hormonal factors affected tendons
17-year-old male, rugby player, traumatic dislocation, shoulder reduced in emergency, painful restriction in movement, progressive weakness, X-ray clear	Positive apprehension test (pain in 90° shoulder abduction)	Anterior shoulder instability	Structural damage often missed on plain X-ray
	Persistent instability + restricted movement	Bankart lesion (labral tear)	MRI suggested if symptoms persist
	Normal X-ray but MRI confirms labral tear – secondary care referral		Needs surgical repair
60-year-old female, history of breast cancer, three months of right arm pain, one year post chemotherapy and radiotherapy	Unexplained unilateral arm pain	Referred non-MSK pain	Urgent red flag due to cancer history
	Cancer history, atypical pain pattern		
X-ray shows shadow – unclear	MRI imaging: Pancoast tumour	Pancoast tumour	Referral to oncology, urgent suspected cancer pathway referral
80-year-old female, diagnosed with polymyalgia rheumatica (PMR), on long-term low-dose steroids – tapering dose of 5 mg, presents with acute and severe shoulder pain, unable to lift arm	Pain with shoulder elevation	Steroid-induced AVN of the shoulder	Risk factor: long-term corticosteroids
	Sudden worsening of pains		Age and PMR are compounding factors
	X-ray shows avascular necrosis (AVN)		Refer for orthopaedic evaluation, emergency referral

Abbreviations: MRI, magnetic resonance imaging; MSK, musculoskeletal; ROM, range of motion.

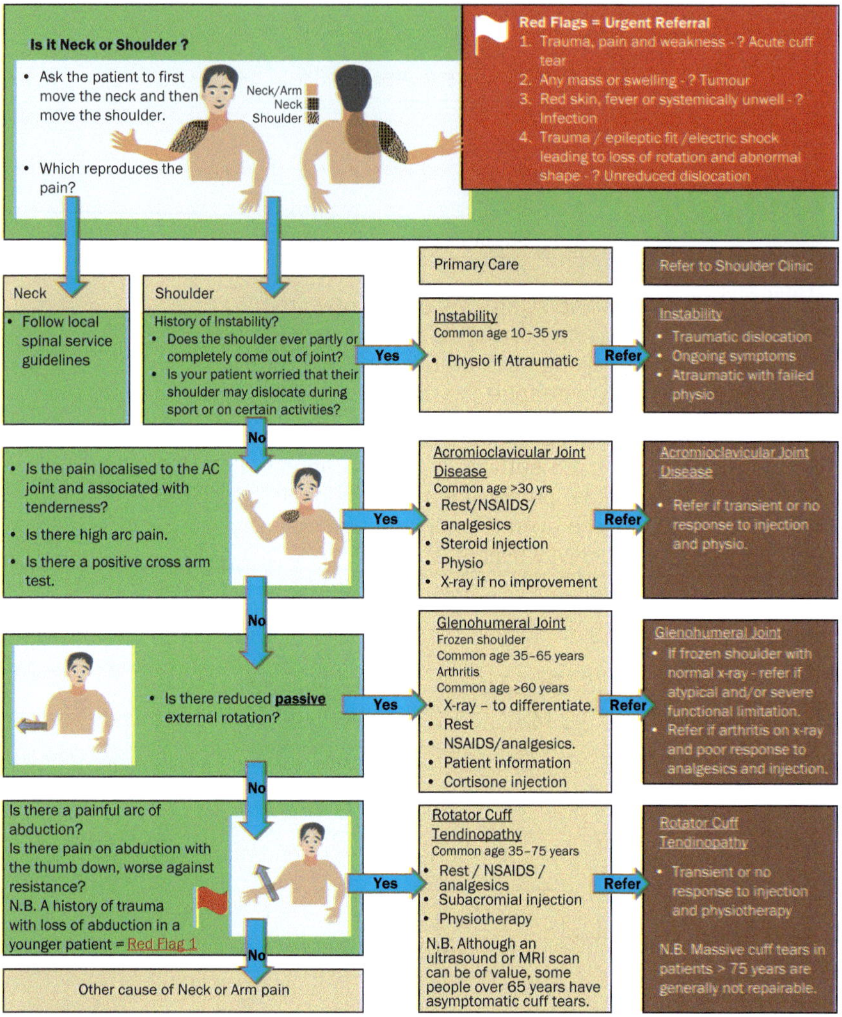

Figure 6.2 Special tests for shoulder problems. Source: British Elbow and Shoulder Society (2023) and British Orthopaedic Association (2022).

Management Strategies for Shoulder Conditions

Conservative Management: Physiotherapy Referral

- **Education and activity modification** – Perform aggravating movements within limitations.

- **Physiotherapy** – Rotator cuff and upper body strengthening, mobility exercises.
- **Pain relief** – NSAIDs, paracetamol, corticosteroid injections (Wang et al., 2017).

Surgical Management (For Severe Cases)

- **Arthroscopic rotator cuff repair** – For full-thickness tears in some cases.
- **Shoulder arthroplasty/replacement** – For end-stage osteoarthritis (Papalia et al., 2020).
- **Stabilisation surgery** – For recurrent instability (Longo et al., 2011).

Key Takeaways

Clinical Red Flags and Diagnostic Approach

Red flag symptoms, such as signs of infection, malignancy or neurological deficits, necessitate urgent investigation and should not be overlooked (NICE, 2023a).

Imaging and Diagnosis

Magnetic resonance imaging is advised for the assessment of soft tissue injuries when symptoms do not improve with conservative management. X-ray imaging remains the first-line investigation for identifying fractures, calcific tendonitis and arthritis (Lewis et al., 2015).

Conservative Management

Most non-traumatic shoulder conditions respond well to early physiotherapy and conservative treatment strategies.

Frozen Shoulder Diagnosis

A diagnosis of frozen shoulder is confirmed when there are notable restrictions and pain during both passive and active external rotation movements of the shoulder.

Soft Tissue Recovery and Rehabilitation

It is important to recognise that soft tissue conditions often require a longer period to recover. Movements, especially progressive loading exercises, carried out within the patient's pain limits are recommended to facilitate improvement.

CHAPTER 7

The Elbow

Introduction

The elbow functions as a hinge joint, permitting movements such as flexion and extension. In addition to these, it allows for pronation and supination, which are essential for the rotation of the forearm. The elbow is integral to the overall function of the upper limb, facilitating a wide range of daily activities. Disorders that affect the elbow can result in pain, reduced range of motion, stiffness and significant impairment in function, thereby impacting a person's ability to perform routine tasks (Standring, 2021). Common conditions seen in primary care are listed in Table 7.1 and red flags to be vigilant of listed in Table 7.2.

Table 7.1 Common elbow conditions.

Condition	Cause	Symptoms	Investigations	Management
Lateral epicondylalgia (tennis elbow)	Overuse, repetitive wrist extension activities Degenerative tendon Inflammatory condition – axial spondyloarthropathy	Lateral elbow pain, weak grip, tenderness over the lateral epicondyle Resisted wrist extension and supination – painful	Clinical diagnosis Ultrasound if intervention is required	Conservative management – activity modification, elbow support, physiotherapy, referral if not better with the above advice NSAIDs (topical)*, shockwave therapy intervention if conservative management fails – referral to secondary care (Coombes et al., 2015)

(*Continued*)

Table 7.1 *(Continued)*

Condition	Cause	Symptoms	Investigations	Management
Medial epicondylalgia (golfer's elbow)	Repetitive wrist flexion activities Overuse Degenerative tendons Inflammatory condition – axial spondyloarthropathy	Medial elbow pain, reduced grip strength Medial epicondyle tenderness Resisted wrist flexion and pronation – painful	Clinical diagnosis Ultrasound if persistent and intervention is required	Conservative management – activity modification, elbow support, physiotherapy referral if not better with the above advice NSAIDs* (topical), shockwave therapy and intervention if conservative management fails – referral to secondary care (Singh et al., 2020)
Olecranon bursitis	Trauma, prolonged pressure, infection, gout	Posterior elbow swelling, tenderness, redness, inflammation	Clinical diagnosis	Rest, ice, compression, NSAIDs*, antibiotics if infected (Blackwell et al., 2014)
Cubital tunnel syndrome	Ulnar nerve compression at the elbow Trauma/injury Repetitive movements Constant pressure on posterior elbow	Numbness, tingling in the ring/little finger, weak grip Tinel's test – tapping under medial epicondyle reproduces paraesthesia, confirms cubital tunnel syndrome	Nerve conduction studies and MRI if required via secondary referral to consultant	Elbow support, referral to physiotherapy for nerve gliding exercises, corticosteroid injection or surgery, secondary referral for surgery if severe symptoms persist (Burahee et al., 2021)
Radial tunnel syndrome	Radial nerve compression due to trauma/ injury, repetitive movements, constant pressure	Deep forearm pain, weakness, paraesthesia	Nerve conduction studies and MRI if required via secondary referral to consultant	Referral to physiotherapy, NSAIDs*, surgical decompression if symptoms persist (Milewski et al., 2019)

Condition	Cause	Symptoms	Investigations	Management
Elbow dislocation	Trauma – falling on the outstretched hand (FOOSH injury)	Severe pain, swelling, tenderness, deformity, loss of function, weakness	X-ray – first line of investigation CT if needed via secondary care referral	Fracture clinic referral – closed reduction, splinting, physiotherapy referral to improve movement and strength (Josefsson et al., 2018)
Osteoarthritis (elbow OA)	Cartilage degeneration, secondary to trauma/injury Age related Overuse Insidious	Stiffness, crepitus, pain, limited range of motion	X-ray (joint space narrowing, osteophytes) – first-line investigation	NSAIDs* (topical) Physiotherapy referral, total elbow replacement if symptoms are severe and persist (Papalia et al., 2020)

*NSAIDs – if allowed/tolerated or start with paracetamol.

Abbreviations: CT, computed tomography; MRI, magnetic resonance imaging; NSAID, non-steroidal anti-inflammatory drug.

Table 7.2 Red flags in elbow disorders.

Red flag	Potential serious condition	Immediate action
Sudden-onset elbow pain with swelling, fever	Septic arthritis	Referral to emergency Urgent joint aspiration, intravenous antibiotics (Mathews et al., 2010)
Persistent non-mechanical pain, unremitting night pain, unexplained weight loss, loss of appetite, history of cancer	Malignancy, metastases	MRI via the urgent suspected cancer pathway (Armstrong et al., 2017)
Acute pain post trauma with or without a deformity	Fracture or dislocation	X-ray – first line of investigation, orthopaedic referral if symptoms persist (Josefsson et al., 2018)

(*Continued*)

Table 7.2 (*Continued*)

Red flag	Potential serious condition	Immediate action
Neurological symptoms (weak grip, numbness, muscle wasting), muscle atrophy	Ulnar/radial nerve entrapment, cervical radiculopathy, neurological disorders such as amyotrophic lateral sclerosis (ALS)	Conservative management – physiotherapy referral Secondary referral – MRI and nerve conduction studies if symptoms persist (Burahee et al., 2021)

Abbreviations: MRI, magnetic resonance imaging.

Anatomy of the Elbow

The elbow joint consists of the following (Figure 7.1).

- **Humeroulnar joint** – Primary hinge movement (flexion/extension).
- **Humeroradial joint** – Assists in pronation/supination.
- **Proximal radioulnar joint** – Enables forearm rotation.
- **Ligaments** – Medial collateral ligament (MCL), lateral collateral ligament (LCL) and annular ligament for stability (Standring, 2021).

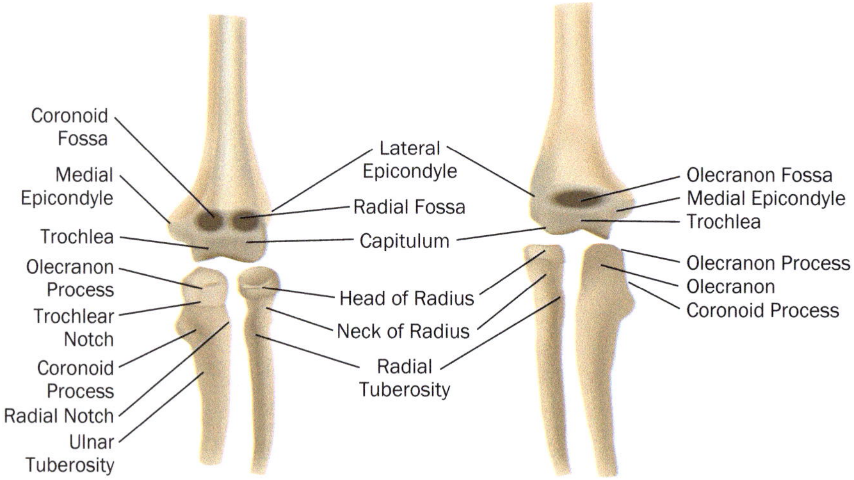

Figure 7.1 Elbow anatomy.

Assessment Approach for Elbow Disorders

Clinical Examination

- **Observation** – Swelling, deformity, muscle wasting, anatomical deviations.
- **Palpation** – Medial and lateral epicondyles, olecranon, radial head.
- **Range of motion (ROM)** – Flexion, extension, supination, pronation (Singh et al., 2020).

Special Tests

Special test for elbow disorders, listed below in Table 7.3.

Table 7.3 Special tests for elbow conditions.

Test	Condition	Positive finding
Cozen's test	Tennis elbow	Pain with resisted wrist extension (Coombes et al., 2015)
Mill's test	Tennis elbow	Pain with passive wrist extension (Milewski et al., 2019)
Golfer's elbow	Golfer's elbow	Pain with resisted wrist flexion
Tinel's sign	Cubital tunnel syndrome	Tingling over ulnar nerve under medial epicondyle (Burahee et al., 2021)
Varus/valgus stress test	Ligament injury	Passive stress on medial or lateral side of the elbow joint in full extension by examiner. Instability or pain with passive stretch to elbow joint confirms ligament injury (Armstrong et al., 2017)

Source: British Elbow and Shoulder Society.

Management Strategies for Elbow Conditions

Conservative Management

- **Education and activity modification** – Perform aggravating movements within limitations.
- **Physiotherapy advice** – Strengthening, mobility exercises for elbow, arm and upper body.
- **Pain relief** – NSAIDs, paracetamol, corticosteroid injections in certain conditions (Coombes et al., 2015).

Surgical Management (For Severe Cases)

- **Arthroscopic debridement** – For severe OA.
- **Ligament reconstruction (Tommy John surgery)** – For UCL injuries (Singh et al., 2020).
- **Nerve decompression surgery** – For cubital tunnel or radial tunnel syndrome (Burahee et al., 2021).

Key Takeaways

Overview of Elbow Joint Pathologies

The elbow joint is particularly susceptible to overuse injuries, as well as syndromes resulting from nerve compression. These conditions are frequently seen in individuals who engage in repetitive arm movements, placing ongoing stress on the structures around the elbow joint.

Red Flags and Urgent Considerations

It is crucial to be vigilant for red flags when assessing elbow complaints (Table 7.4). The presence of infection, malignancy or severe trauma should prompt immediate investigation and intervention, as these conditions can have serious consequences if not addressed promptly (NICE, 2023a).

Management of Common Elbow Conditions

Tennis elbow, or lateral epicondylitis, often resolves without invasive treatment if activities are modified. However, in cases where symptoms persist, further intervention may be warranted. Early implementation of physiotherapy and conservative strategies is generally effective for most non-traumatic elbow conditions, helping to restore function and reduce discomfort.

Olecranon Bursitis

Sudden, insidious onset of olecranon bursitis can sometimes be linked to underlying conditions such as gout. For further detail on the relationship between gout and bursitis, refer to Chapter 12.

Table 7.4 Elbow clinical scenarios: pattern recognition and red flags.

Clinical scenario	Key clinical tests/ observations	Likely diagnosis/ pattern	Red flags/ additional considerations
1. 42-year-old desk worker male, plays squash and tennis, complains of elbow pain with right-sided use of mouse and DIY activities	Tender lateral epicondyle Pain on resisted wrist extension Worse with gripping movement Localised to lateral elbow	Lateral epicondylitis (tennis elbow)	Conservative management – physiotherapy referral Activity modification advice Ergonomic assessment advice

Clinical scenario	Key clinical tests/ observations	Likely diagnosis/ pattern	Red flags/ additional considerations
2. 55-year-old male, smoker 10/day, drinker, two pints of beer every day, hypercholesteraemia, complains of sudden elbow pain, sedentary job and lifestyle	Red, hot, swollen elbow on observation Painful movements Often monoarticular	Gout (olecranon bursitis/intra-articular gout)	Classic presentation in metabolic syndrome Check urate, after six weeks of acute flare Responds to NSAIDs and colchicine Rule out infection (aspiration if infected)
3. 36-year-old female, PhD student, reported numbness on inner elbow for past one month, has noticed grip muscle weakness	Numbness 4th/5th digits Tinel's at cubital tunnel Elbow flexion test positive ↓ Grip strength	Cubital tunnel syndrome (ulnar nerve entrapment)	Desk-related compression of ulnar nerve Activity modification Physiotherapy referral Neurosurgery referral if symptoms persist
4. 46-year-old male reported pain distal to lateral epicondyle, ↑ with supination and gripping, no numbness	Tender lateral forearm Resisted supination painful No sensory loss Often misdiagnosed as tennis elbow	Radial tunnel syndrome (posterior interosseous nerve entrapment)	Differentiate from lateral epicondylitis Activity modification Physiotherapy referral – neural glides Consider imaging referral via secondary care if symptoms are persistent

Abbreviations: NSAID, non-steroidal anti-inflammatory drug.

CHAPTER 8

The Wrist and Hand

Introduction

The wrist and hand are intricate anatomical regions, specifically developed to facilitate dexterity, strength and precise motor control. Owing to the significant functional demands placed upon them, these structures are particularly vulnerable to various forms of trauma, repetitive strain injuries and age-related degenerative changes (Standring, 2021). Common conditions are listed in Table 8.1 and red flags to be vigilant for in Table 8.2.

Table 8.1 Common wrist and hand conditions.

	Cause	Symptoms	Investigations	Management
Carpal tunnel syndrome (CTS)	Median nerve compression, diabetes, overuse, metabolic changes, age related Pregnancy related Hormonal changes	Numbness, tingling (thumb, index, middle finger), night waking due to paraesthesia	Nerve conduction studies, MRI via secondary care referral if not improving Clinical diagnosis	Conservative treatment – night splint, corticosteroid injections if thenar eminence is not wasted, wrist extension stretches Severe cases – carpal tunnel release (Atroshi et al., 2019)

(Continued)

Table 8.1 (*Continued*)

	Cause	Symptoms	Investigations	Management
De Quervain's tenosynovitis	Overuse of thumb abductor and extensor tendons Pregnancy, overuse, repetitive loading for e.g. desk work	Radial-sided wrist pain at base of the thumb, pain with lifting, in radial deviation	Finkelstein's test – clinical diagnosis, ultrasound via secondary care referral if not improving	Activity modification, grip strengthening, de Quervain's splint, NSAIDs* (topical), corticosteroid injections – ultrasound guided via secondary care (Wolf et al., 2009)
Trigger finger (stenosing tenosynovitis)	Tendon sheath inflammation, overuse, age related, metabolic changes, hormonal changes	Finger locking, pain, clicking sensation at base of the metacarpals Catching sensation Nodule at the base of metacarpal	Clinical diagnosis, locking can be seen with finger flexion, usually ring finger and thumb are common sites	Conservative management – splint, trigger finger release massage, corticosteroid injections, surgical release if persistent (Makkouk et al., 2008)
Wrist and finger osteoarthritis (OA)	Cartilage degeneration, age related, trauma, insidious Rheumatological conditions	Stiffness, pain, reduced grip strength, OA nodes on hands and fingers – Heberden's and Bouchard's	X-ray (joint space narrowing, osteophytes)	NSAIDs* (topical), wrist support, movements and strength exercise advice, joint fusion or replacement if severe symptoms persist (Zhang et al., 2009)
Scaphoid fracture	FOOSH injury (fall on outstretched hand), osteoporotic fractures	Radial wrist pain, snuffbox tenderness	X-ray (initial), MRI/CT via secondary care referral if X-ray is negative and symptoms persist	Thumb spica support, thumb stretches and strength advice, surgical intervention if severe symptoms persist (Dias et al., 2016)

	Cause	Symptoms	Investigations	Management
Distal radius fracture (Colles' fracture)	FOOSH injury	Wrist deformity, pain, swelling Bruising	X-ray (dorsal displacement)	Fracture clinic referral, cast immobilisation, surgical fixation via orthopaedic referral if unstable (Bentohami et al., 2014)
Smith's fracture	Fall on a flexed wrist (opposite to Colles' fracture)	Acute wrist pain Swelling Bruising Tenderness	X-ray first line of management CT via secondary care referral if symptoms persist	Fracture clinic referral Closed reduction Open reduction and internal fixation (ORIF) Physiotherapy referral (Schroeder and Varacallo, 2024)
Dupuytren's contracture	Progressive thickening and shortening of palmar fascia affecting ring and little fingers Males commonly affected Genetic disorder Smoking Diabetes Alcoholism Epilepsy medication Manual workers Can be bilateral	Painless nodules in the palm Cord formation in flexor tendons Finger flexion deformity Cannot put hands flat on the table (tabletop test) Difficulty and catching in daily activities	Clinical diagnosis Ultrasound via secondary care referral only if unsure about the diagnosis	Conservative management – early disease Exercise advice to extend fingers If the contracture >30° then refer onwards to hand surgeon for fasciotomy (BMJ Best Practice, 2023)

*NSAIDs – if allowed or prescribe paracetamol.

Abbreviations: CT, computed tomography; MRI, magnetic resonance imaging; NSAID, non-steroidal anti-inflammatory drug.

Table 8.2 Red flags in wrist and hand disorders.

Red flag	Potential serious condition	Immediate action
Acute wrist pain with swelling, fever/chills/existing infection	Septic arthritis, flexor tenosynovitis	Refer to emergency Urgent aspiration, IV antibiotics (Mathews et al., 2008; 2010)
Persistent, non-mechanical pain, night pain, unexplained weight loss >5% body weight in the past 6–12 months, history of cancer, malaise, lumps or unusual swelling	Malignancy, metastases	MRI via urgent suspected cancer pathway (Zhang et al., 2009)
Wrist deformity post trauma, fall	Fracture, dislocation	X-ray Fracture clinic referral, orthopaedic referral for surgical intervention (Bentohami et al., 2014)
Severe nerve pain, loss of function, atrophy, paraesthesia, muscle wasting	Nerve entrapment syndromes, e.g. carpal tunnel syndrome	Nerve conduction studies via secondary care referral, wrist support, surgical release if needed via orthopaedic referral (Atroshi et al., 2019)

Abbreviations: IV, intravenous; MRI, magnetic resonance imaging.

Anatomy of the Wrist and Hand

The wrist consists of the following aspects (Figure 8.1).

- **Radiocarpal joint** – Allows flexion, extension, radial and ulnar deviation.
- **Midcarpal joint** – Contributes to wrist motion.
- **Distal radioulnar joint (DRUJ)** – Responsible for forearm rotation.

The hand consists of the following aspects.

- **Carpals, metacarpals and phalanges** – Supporting grip strength.
- **Intrinsic and extrinsic muscles** – Controlling fine and gross motor function.
- **Tendons, ligaments and nerves** – Providing stability and sensation (Standring 2021).

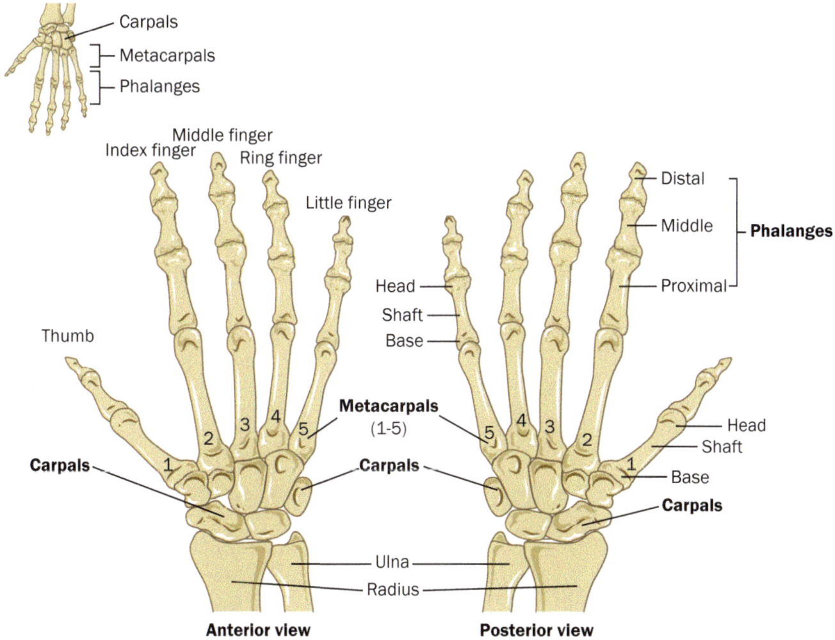

Figure 8.1 Wrist and hand anatomy.

Assessment Approach for Wrist and Hand Disorders

Clinical Examination

- **Observation** – Swelling, deformity, muscle atrophy, anatomical variations.
- **Palpation** – Snuffbox tenderness (scaphoid fracture), joint tenderness.
- **Range of motion (ROM)** – Wrist flexion, extension, grip strength (Wolf et al., 2009).

Special Tests

Table 8.3 Special tests for wrist and hand conditions.

Test	Condition	Positive finding
Phalen's test – patient keeps backs of hands placed together, fingers down, hold for 30 seconds. Test is positive with onset of paraesthesia	Carpal tunnel syndrome	Numbness in median nerve distribution (Atroshi et al., 2019)

(Continued)

Table 8.3 *(Continued)*

Test	Condition	Positive finding
Tinel's sign – tapping on anterior wrist crease with palmar surface facing upwards. Test is positive with onset of paraesthesia	Carpal tunnel syndrome	Tingling over median nerve distribution (Makkouk et al., 2008)
Tabletop test – inability to place hand flat on a table. Test is positive	Dupuytren's contracture	Flexion contracture of little and ring finger in severe cases (BMJ Best Practice, 2023)
Finkelstein's test – make a fist with thumb inside the palm, and bend the wrist towards little finger. Test is positive with onset of pain	De Quervain's tenosynovitis	Pain with ulnar deviation and thumb flexion (Wolf et al., 2009)

Management Strategies for Wrist and Hand Conditions

Conservative Management

- **Education and activity modification** – Reducing repetitive strain, pace activities.
- **Physiotherapy/hand therapy** – Strengthening, mobility exercises for wrist, hand, grip, splints and/or supports.
- **Pain relief** – NSAIDs (topical), paracetamol; corticosteroid injections via secondary care referral are unavailable in primary care (Zhang et al., 2009).

Surgical Management (For Severe Cases)

- **Carpal tunnel release** – For persistent carpal tunnel syndrome.
- **Wrist arthroplasty** – For severe OA.
- **Thumb replacement** – For severe carpometacarpal joint OA.
- **Scaphoid ORIF (open reduction internal fixation)** – For displaced fractures (Dias et al., 2016).

Key Takeaways

Wrist and hand disorders are prevalent, owing to the high functional demands placed on these structures and the frequency of trauma to the area.

Urgent Red Flags

Certain presentations, such as suspected infection, malignancy or fractures, should prompt immediate referral for specialist assessment (Table 8.4) (NICE, 2023a).

Imaging and Diagnosis

Magnetic resonance imaging plays a crucial role in the assessment of soft tissue injuries, offering detailed visualisation that guides management. For fractures and arthritis, an X-ray remains the initial investigation of choice. In cases where a scaphoid fracture is suspected but not apparent on X-ray, a CT scan should be arranged to confirm or exclude the diagnosis (Bentohami et al., 2014).

Conservative Management

Early physiotherapy and conservative treatment approaches are generally effective for the majority of non-traumatic wrist and hand conditions. Topical NSAIDs are indicated for wrist and hand osteoarthritis (NICE, 2025).

Consideration of Rheumatological Conditions

Sudden, insidious inflammation affecting the hands and fingers may suggest an underlying rheumatological condition. Further information on this can be found in Chapter 12.

Table 8.4 Wrist and hand clinical scenarios: pattern recognition and red flags.

Clinical scenario	Key clinical tests/ observations	Likely diagnosis/ pattern	Red flags/additional considerations
1. 43-year-old female art curator, loves knitting, reported painful waking with pins and needles for past two months, weakness in hand and grip muscles	Numbness in thumb, index, middle fingers Positive Phalen's and Tinel's Night symptoms common Decreased thenar eminence strength (if chronic, wasting is noted)	Carpal tunnel syndrome (CTS)	Median nerve compression Night splinting Ergonomic mouse advice + nerve glides via physiotherapy referral Corticosteroid injection (ultrasound guided, if possible, via secondary care referral) Nerve conduction studies if no change in symptoms and requires surgical intervention if thenar eminence wasting noted

(Continued)

Table 8.4 *(Continued)*

Clinical scenario	Key clinical tests/ observations	Likely diagnosis/ pattern	Red flags/additional considerations
2. 48-year-old female, baker, ulnar-sided wrist pain after rowing competition, struggles with gripping pen, spoons and ladles	Increased pain with ulnar deviation movements Tender over triangular fibrocartilage complex (TFCC) region Decreased grip strength Clicking sensation with wrist and hand movements Experiencing pain during ulnar deviation with a closed fist is considered a positive sign for TFCC injury	TFCC tear	Often traumatic or overuse MRI or wrist arthrogram via orthopaedic hand consultant referral if persistent Splinting or ortho referral if severe
3. 64-year-old female, seamstress, struggling with holding toothbrush, knife/fork, dressing, finger is catching	Palpable nodule Finger clicks or locks Painful extension of finger after locking	Trigger finger	Common in repetitive hand use, age, hormonal changes, metabolic factors – diabetes, thyroid, etc. Rest, splinting, steroid injection if available in primary care or secondary care referral Surgical release if chronic and unresolved symptoms
4. 22-year-old male cyclist, falls on outstretched hand (FOOSH), swelling, bruising, can't grip/lift with this hand, struggling with typing	Tender anatomical snuffbox Pain with axial thumb compression Decreased grip and hand muscle strength	Scaphoid fracture	Missed fractures can lead to avascular necrosis Immobilise even if X-ray normal for missed fractures Repeat imaging in 10–14 days or MRI via orthopaedic referral

CHAPTER 9

The Hip, Pelvis and Sacroiliac Joint

Introduction

The hip, pelvis and sacroiliac joint (SIJ) play a vital role in supporting load bearing, facilitating mobility and transmitting force between the axial skeleton and the lower appendicular skeleton. When dysfunction occurs in any of these areas, it can result in significant pain, disturbances in gait and a marked reduction in functional capacity. Such impairments may have a considerable impact on daily activities and overall quality of life (Standring, 2021). Common conditions affecting hip and SIJ seen in primary care are listed in Table 9.1 and red flags to be vigilant for are shown in Table 9.2.

Table 9.1 Common hip, pelvis and SIJ conditions.

Condition	Cause	Symptoms	Investigations	Management
Osteoarthritis (hip OA)	Cartilage degeneration Insidious Trauma Overuse Metabolic factors Obesity Rheumatology conditions (information in Chapter 12)	Groin pain, stiffness, reduced range of motion in hip movements, painful walking, steps, standing, rising from sitting position	Clinical diagnosis for >45 years X-ray (joint space narrowing, osteophytes)	Physiotherapy referral, mobility and activity modification exercises, NSAIDs*, weight reduction advice, hip replacement if severe and symptoms persist (Hunter and Bierma-Zeinstra, 2022)

(Continued)

Table 9.1 *(Continued)*

Condition	Cause	Symptoms	Investigations	Management
Femoro-acetabular impingement (FAI)	Abnormal femoral or acetabular morphology Congenital hip disorders Overuse Trauma/injury	Hip/groin pain, clicking, reduced range of motion Painful weight bearing Walking, jumping, squatting Hip flexion, abduction and lateral rotation pains (FABER test) – painful	X-ray – to rule out trauma (cam/pincer deformity), MRI for labral changes via secondary care orthopaedic referral	Physiotherapy referral, activity modification advice, orthopaedic surgery if required (Griffin et al., 2016)
Hip labral tear	Trauma, repetitive strain injuries Osteoarthritis	Anterior hip pain, clicking, instability Hip flexion, abduction and lateral rotation pains (FABER test) – painful	MRI arthrogram (gold standard) via secondary care orthopaedic referral	Physiotherapy referral, activity modification advice, hip arthroscopy if symptomatic and painful (Nepple et al., 2018)
Sacroiliac joint (SIJ) dysfunction	Trauma, overuse, pregnancy, inflammatory conditions	Low back/ buttock pain, pain with prolonged standing, pain when walking or coming up or down stairs	SIJ provocative tests, MRI for inflammatory conditions	Physiotherapy referral, Pilates exercise advice, pain referral for injections if symptoms persist (Vleeming et al., 2012)
Greater trochanteric pain syndrome/ lateral hip pain	Overuse, age, hormonal changes, metabolic changes, insidious onset, OA Degenerative tendons	Side-lying pains, single leg stance pains, tender over greater trochanter, painful walking, climbing steps	Clinical diagnosis; painful resisted hip abduction is positive	Topical ice pack 10–15 min 2–3/ day advice, no cross-leg sitting, physiotherapy referral for tendon loading exercises, injections only if no better with conservative management

*NSAIDs – if allowed or start with paracetamol.

Abbreviations: MRI, magnetic resonance imaging; NSAID, non-steroidal anti-inflammatory drug.

Table 9.2 Red flags in hip and SIJ disorders.

Red flag	Potential serious condition	Immediate action
Acute hip pain with inability to bear weight, leg externally rotated, limp Due to falls, osteoporosis, trauma/injury	Hip fracture	Urgent X-ray, MRI if needed via orthopaedic referral (Royal Osteoporosis Society, 2022), MRI if occult fracture suspected Surgical fixation (dynamic hip screw, total hip replacement), physiotherapy referral, osteoporosis management (Royal Osteoporosis Society, 2022)
Progressive hip pain with unremitting night pain, unexplained weight loss >5% of body weight in the past 6–12 months, history of cancer	Malignancy, metastatic disease	MRI, urgent suspected cancer referral (Hunter and Bierma-Zeinstra, 2022)
Sudden-onset hip pain with fever/chills, systemic symptoms (feeling unwell, recent infection)	Septic arthritis	Urgent joint aspiration via emergency referral, IV antibiotics (Mathews et al., 2010)
Persistent groin pain in young athletes, difficulty weight bearing	Stress fracture (femoral neck)	Emergency referral MRI, activity modification, orthopaedic referral (Nepple et al., 2018)
Progressive hip pain, reduced range of movement – due to risk factors such as corticosteroid use, alcohol, trauma, insidious, age related	Avascular necrosis (AVN) of the hip	X-ray in primary care, MRI, urgent emergency referral NSAIDs*, bisphosphonates, core decompression, total hip replacement if severe (Mont et al., 2015)

*NSAIDs – if allowed or start with paracetamol.

Abbreviations: IV, intravenous; MRI, magnetic resonance imaging.

Anatomy of the Hip, Pelvis and Sacroiliac Joint

- **Hip joint** – A ball-and-socket synovial joint, designed for stability and mobility.
- **Pelvis** – Composed of the ilium, ischium and pubis, forming the pelvic ring.
- **Sacroiliac joint (SIJ)** – A strong yet less mobile joint, connecting the sacrum to the ilium, aiding in force distribution (Vleeming et al., 2012) (Figure 9.1).

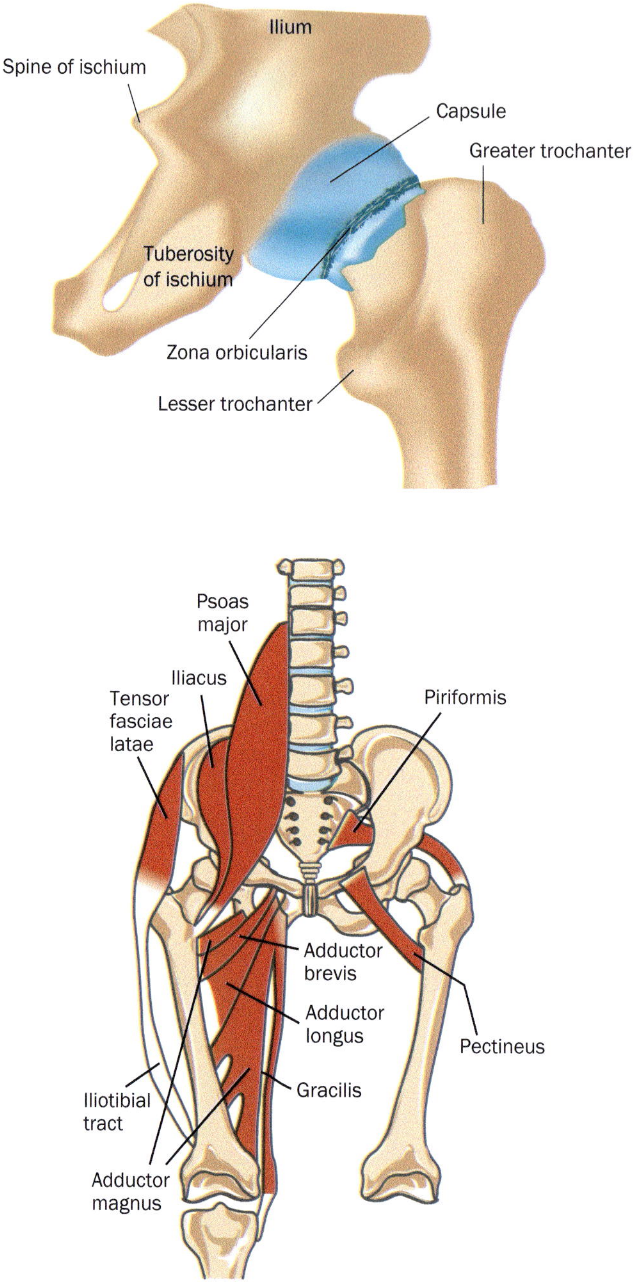

Figure 9.1 Hip and SIJ anatomy.

Assessment Approach for Hip, Pelvis and Sacroiliac Joint Disorders

Clinical Examination

- **Observation** – Gait analysis, leg length discrepancy, anatomical deviations, check for redness, swelling, bruises, deformity.
- **Palpation** – Bony landmarks, soft tissue tenderness, muscle tightness.
- **Range of motion (ROM)** – Flexion, extension, abduction, adduction, internal/external rotation (Griffin et al., 2016).

Special Tests

Table 9.3 Special tests in hip and SIJ conditions.

Test	Condition	Positive finding
FABER test – flexion, abduction and external rotation of hip in supine	SIJ dysfunction, hip osteoarthritis (OA), femoro-acetabular impingement (FAI)	Reproduces posterior hip pain (Vleeming et al., 2012)
FADIR test – flexion, adduction and internal rotation of hip in supine	Femoro-acetabular impingement	Groin pain (Nepple et al., 2018)
Trendelenburg test – when standing on one leg, hip drop is positive	Hip abductor weakness commonly seen in neurological disorders or severe joint and muscle conditions	Contralateral hip drop (Hunter and Bierma-Zeinstra, 2022)
Scour test – hip joint circumduction in supine	Hip intra-articular pathology – OA	Positive if painful
Single-leg squat test and tenderness over greater trochanter	Pain in weight-bearing leg	Greater trochanteric pain syndrome (GTPS) Lateral hip pain/gluteal tendinopathy (Mellor et al. 2018)

Management Strategies for Hip, Pelvis and Sacroiliac Joint Conditions

Conservative Management

- **Education and activity modification** – Advice about pacing and performing aggravating movements within pain limits.
- **Physiotherapy referral** – Strengthening, mobility exercises for back, core and legs.

- **Pain relief** – NSAIDs (topical/oral), paracetamol, intra-articular corticosteroid injections under ultrasound guidance via secondary care (Hunter and Bierma-Zeinstra, 2022)

Surgical Management (for Severe Cases)

- **Hip arthroscopy** – For FAI, labral tears.
- **Total hip replacement (THR)** – For severe hip osteoarthritis and poor quality of life (Mont et al., 2015).
- **SIJ fusion** – For chronic, refractory SIJ dysfunction (Vleeming et al., 2012).

Key Takeaways

Dysfunctions affecting the hip, pelvis and SIJ are frequently encountered in clinical practice. However, it is crucial to distinguish these musculoskeletal conditions from more serious underlying pathologies. This differentiation ensures that life- or limb-threatening conditions are not missed.

Identification of Red Flags

Certain clinical features serve as red flags and should prompt urgent further investigation (Table 9.4). These include persistent night pain, the presence of systemic symptoms or a sudden, acute inability to bear weight. Recognising these signs is essential to avoid delays in diagnosing potentially serious causes, as recommended by national guidelines (NICE, 2023a).

Role of Imaging

Magnetic resonance imaging (MRI) is a vital tool in the early detection of specific conditions such as avascular necrosis (AVN), labral tears and stress fractures (Nepple et al., 2018).

Conservative Management

For the majority of non-traumatic hip, pelvis and SIJ conditions, early engagement with physiotherapy and conservative management strategies is effective. These approaches may include targeted exercises, education and activity modification aimed at reducing pain and improving function.

Greater Trochanteric Pain Syndrome

A common presentation is pain lying on one side, pain with going up or down steps and discomfort during single-leg stance, often localised to the lateral hip, commonly seen with hormonal changes. These symptoms are suggestive of greater trochanteric pain syndrome. Management should be conservative, focusing on progressive loading exercises, physiotherapy input and the possible use of shockwave therapy to facilitate recovery.

Table 9.4 Hip clinical scenarios: pattern recognition and red flags.

Clinical scenario	Key clinical tests/ observations	Likely diagnosis/ pattern	Red flags/additional considerations
1. 43-year-old female, yoga teacher, right hip pain, can't sleep on right side, struggles with stairs, struggling with sleep, regular runner	Tender greater trochanter Pain with single-leg stance and squat Positive resisted abduction	Greater trochanteric pain syndrome	Load-related overuse Educate on sleep/ stairs Progressive loading Physiotherapy referral if symptoms worsen
2. 19-year-old male gymnast, acute right hip pain with training, sudden onset, unable to bear weight on right side	Pain on passive ROM Positive FADIR Guarded hip posture Reduced mobility	Intra-articular trauma or avulsion injury	MRI via secondary care referral Rule out labral tear, stress fracture Ortho referral for intervention
3. 56-year-old female, history of breast cancer (15 years ago), hip pain with running, fatigue but no night sweats, no unexplained weight loss within 6–12 months	Non-mechanical pain Proximal femur tenderness Systemic fatigue	Metastases suspected	Cancer history = red flag Urgent MRI via urgent suspected cancer pathway referral Oncology referral
4. 32-year-old female desk worker with six months onset of right hip and groin pain with running and sitting in low chair, weight-bearing hip pains at night	Groin pain, lateral hip pain Clicking and catching sensation Painful limited hip flexion, internal rotation, external rotation	Hip dysplasia	X-ray hip dysplasia MRI labral tear via secondary care referral Physiotherapy referral, activity modification If symptoms worsen, secondary care referral for hip arthroscopy

Abbreviations: MRI, magnetic resonance imaging; ROM, range of motion.

CHAPTER 10

The Knee

Introduction

The knee functions as a hinge joint that is essential for providing both stability and mobility to the lower limb. In addition, it plays a crucial part in absorbing shock during movement. Due to its anatomical structure and the range of activities it supports, the knee is particularly vulnerable to injury, degenerative changes and conditions related to overuse. As a result, knee pain is a common reason for patients to seek care in a primary care setting (Standring, 2021).

The origin of knee pain can be diverse. It may arise from intra-articular structures such as the menisci, ligaments or articular cartilage. Alternatively, pain can result from issues affecting periarticular soft tissues, including tendons and bursae. In some cases, knee pain reflects underlying systemic conditions, such as inflammatory arthritis, infections or malignancy (Hunter and Bierma-Zeinstra, 2022). Common knee conditions seen in primary care are listed in Table 10.1, red flags to be vigilant for are listed in Table 10.2 and assessments for knee conditions are listed in Table 10.3.

Table 10.1 Common knee conditions.

Condition	Cause	Symptoms	Investigations	Management
Osteoarthritis (knee OA)	Cartilage degeneration, overuse, trauma, insidious, weight issues and metabolic causes	Pain, stiffness, crepitus, reduced ROM Muscle weakness, balance issues	Clinical diagnosis – no investigations required X-ray (joint space narrowing, osteophytes) if an intervention is required	Advice – reduce weight, strengthen muscles Physiotherapy referral if not better, NSAIDs* (topical), weight loss, psychosocial support, steroid injections for temporary pain relief and improving quality of life Joint replacement if function is poor (Hunter and Bierma-Zeinstra, 2022)
Meniscal tear	Trauma, degeneration, overuse, sports injury, insidious	Knee joint locking, clicking, joint line tenderness	Secondary care referral – MRI (gold standard), McMurray's test +	Muscle strengthening advice, physiotherapy referral, steroid injections for temporary pain relief, surgical referral if no improvement in function (Beaufils et al., 2017)
Ligament tears	Trauma (pivoting, hyperextension injuries), sports, overuse, trauma, degenerative	Knee joint instability, swelling, giving way, weakness	MRI, Lachman's test (ACL), posterior drawer test (PCL)	Muscle strengthening advice, physiotherapy referral, ACL reconstruction if unstable joint (Ardern et al., 2018)
Patellofemoral pain syndrome (PFPS)/anterior knee pain (AKP)	Patellar orientation, tracking, overuse, muscular dysfunction	Anterior knee pain, worse with stairs, prolonged sitting – cinema sign – pain after prolonged sitting	Clinical diagnosis, MRI via secondary care referral only if atypical symptoms	Activity modification, taping for stability (Willy et al., 2019)

Chondromalacia patellae	Cartilage degeneration Overuse Insidious onset	Anterior knee pain, crepitus, pain with stair climbing	X-ray, MRI via secondary care referral if no improvement seen	Muscle strengthening advice, physiotherapy referral, NSAIDs*, activity modification, steroid injections for temporary pain relief (Crossley et al., 2016)
Bursitis (posterior bursa = Baker's cyst) Housemaid's knee	Swelling and inflammation of knee bursae, due to arthritis, trauma or overuse, insidious	Redness, swelling, inflammation, painful movements, for example kneeling	Clinical diagnosis Ultrasound if not improving	Ice/compression, support, NSAIDS*, steroid injection with or without aspiration in primary care or secondary care
Haemarthrosis	Post surgery, infection, injury, bleeding disorders Degenerative vascular	Painful and reduced movements, redness, inflammation, swelling around the joint, joint instability	X-ray to rule out fracture MRI gold standard via secondary care referral	Ice, compression, joint aspiration, NSAIDS* Steroid injection, arthroscopy/synovectomy via secondary care referral (Papalia et al., 2021)
Patellar tendinopathy/jumper's knee	Overuse, repetitive loading, jumping, squatting and running	Gradual onset of anterior knee pain, localised to patellar tendon	Clinical diagnosis If sinister pathologies suspected, ultrasound and MRI if required, via secondary care referral	Conservative management Activity modification, loading exercises (Theodorou et al., 2023)

*NSAIDs – if allowed or start with paracetamol.

Abbreviations: ACL, anterior cruciate ligament; MRI, magnetic resonance imaging; NSAID, non-steroidal anti-inflammatory drug; PCL, posterior cruciate ligament.

Table 10.2 Red flags and emergency referral criteria for knee disorders.

Red flag	Potential serious condition	Immediate action
Severe pain, rapid swelling after twisting injury, redness, inflammation Locking, weight-bearing issues and weakness	Meniscal tears	Urgent X-ray to rule out fracture Secondary care referral. Urgent MRI via orthopaedic referral (Ardern et al., 2018)
Inability to bear weight, flexion/hyperextension injury – instability in the knee joint, swelling, severe pains, inflammation, redness	Ligament rupture (ACL, PCL, MCL, LCL)	Urgent X-ray to rule out fracture Secondary care referral for MRI – orthopaedic review (Beaufils et al., 2017)
Erythema, warmth, fever with knee pain post systemic/ local infection	Septic arthritis, osteomyelitis	Refer to emergency Emergency joint aspiration, IV antibiotics (Mathews et al., 2010)
Unremitting night pain, unexplained weight loss >5% of body weight in the past 6–12 months, history of cancer, feeling unwell, fatigue, painful weight bearing, lumps	Bone malignancy (osteosarcoma) Soft tissue sarcoma	Urgent imaging via urgent suspected cancer pathway (Hunter and Bierma-Zeinstra, 2022)
Severe pain post injury, swelling, inability to bear weight, post high-velocity trauma (sports, road traffic collision, falls); if popliteal artery is involved then vascular assessment is warranted	Dislocation	Early reduction via referral to fracture clinic/ emergency to avoid compartment syndrome, vascular compromise (Teissier et al., 2019)

Abbreviations: ACL, anterior cruciate ligament; LCL, lateral collateral ligament; MCL, medial collateral ligament; MRI, magnetic resonance imaging; PCL, posterior cruciate ligament.

Knee Assessment Protocol

History Taking

- **Pain location** – Anterior (patellofemoral pain syndrome, chondromalacia patellae), medial/lateral (meniscal, MCL/LCL injuries), posterior (Baker's cyst, hamstring injury).
- **Onset** – Acute (trauma) versus chronic (degenerative, overuse).
- **Character** – Sharp, dull, locking, instability.
- **Aggravating and relieving factors** – Activity, stairs, rest.
- **Systemic symptoms** – Fever, unexplained weight loss, night pain (Hunter and Bierma-Zeinstra, 2022).

Table 10.3 Special tests for knee conditions.

Observation	Palpation	Range of motion (ROM)	Special tests	Result
Swelling, and redness if acute	Joint line tenderness, effusion	Knee joint extension, flexion restrictions	Lachman test – With the patient supine and knee flexed 20–30°, anterior tibial translation indicates ACL laxity	ACL tear (Ardern et al., 2018)
Swelling/ redness if acute	Joint line tenderness, effusion	Knee joint extension, flexion restrictions	McMurray's test – With the patient supine, fully flex the knee, then extend while rotating it internally and externally. Pain indicates a positive result	Meniscal tear (Beaufils et al., 2017)

(*Continued*)

Table 10.3 *(Continued)*

Observation	Palpation	Range of motion (ROM)	Special tests	Result
Patellar malalignment	Patellofemoral joint line tenderness, patellar tracking issues	Knee extension pains, prolonged sitting pains	Patellar grind test (Clarke's test) – With the patient in a supine position, apply inferior compression to the patella while instructing the patient to contract the quadriceps muscle. A positive result is indicated by the presence of pain during this manoeuvre	Patellofemoral pain syndrome (Crossley et al., 2016)
Antalgic gait and giving way	Tenderness and lax joint movement	Laxity	Varus/valgus stress tests – Assess knee stability by applying medial and lateral force; laxity indicates a positive result	MCL/LCL injuries (Willy et al., 2019)

Abbreviations: ACL, anterior cruciate ligament; LCL, lateral collateral ligament; MCL, medial collateral ligament.

Anatomy Overview

The knee joint consists of the following aspects (Figure 10.1).

- **Bones** – Femur, tibia, patella, fibula.
- **Menisci** – Medial and lateral menisci for shock absorption.
- **Ligaments** – ACL, PCL, MCL, LCL for stability.
- **Tendons and muscles** – Quadriceps, hamstrings, patellar tendon.
- **Bursae** – Prepatellar, infrapatellar, pes anserine bursae.
- **Neurovascular structures** – Sciatic nerve, femoral nerve, popliteal artery (Standring 2021).

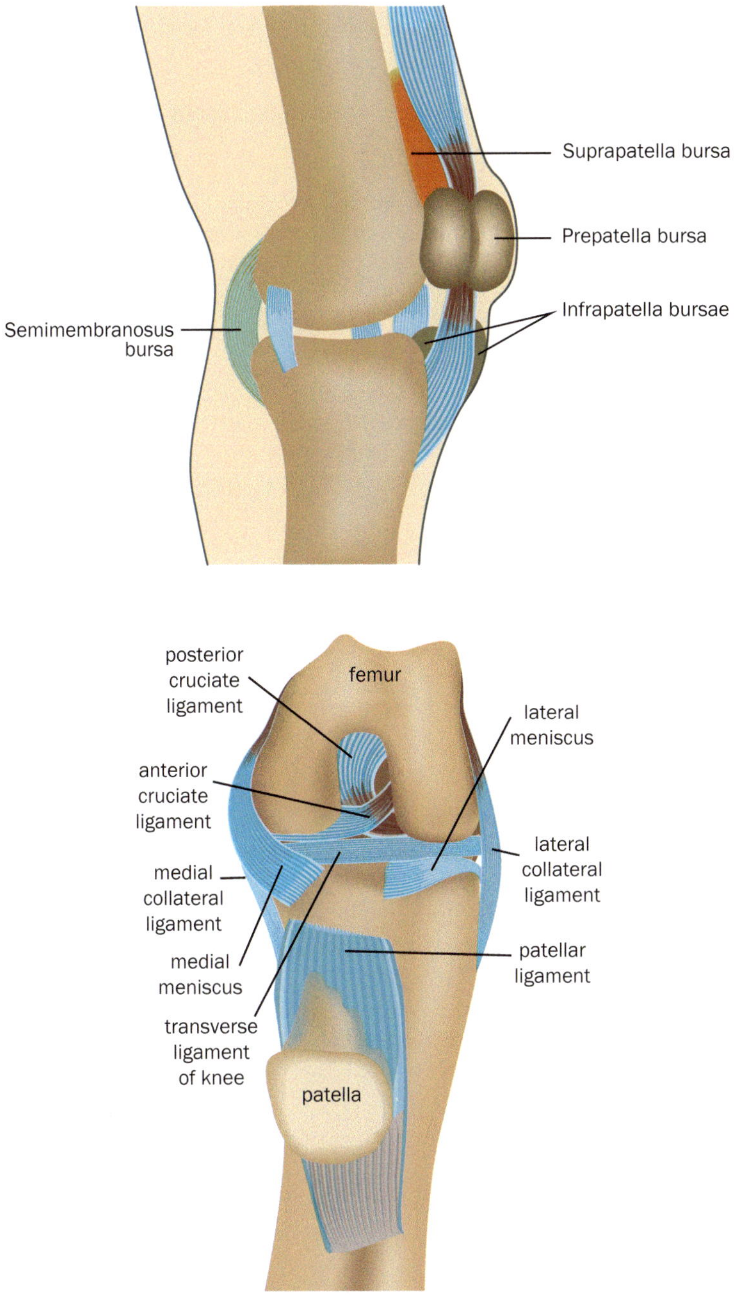

Figure 10.1 Knee anatomy and bursae.

Management Strategies for Knee Conditions

Conservative Management

- **Activity modification and education** – Pacing, recommend weight loss regime, knee support for instability, education, reassurance, psychological support.
- **Physiotherapy referral** – For lower limb strengthening exercises, functional rehabilitation, mobility exercises, education.
- **Pain relief** – NSAIDs, paracetamol, corticosteroid injections for improving quality of life (Hunter and Bierma-Zeinstra, 2022).

Interventional Management (for Refractory Cases)

- **Intra-articular corticosteroid injections** – Knee OA, inflammatory conditions.
- **Surgical referral:**
  - **Total or partial knee replacement (TKR)** – Severe OA.
  - **Arthroscopy** – Meniscal repair, ligament reconstruction.
  - **Osteotomy** – Corrective realignment procedures (Beaufils et al., 2017).

Key Takeaways

Causes of Knee Pain

Knee pain may originate from a variety of sources, including mechanical dysfunctions, inflammatory processes, traumatic events or underlying systemic conditions.

Common Conditions

One prevalent cause of anterior knee pain is chondromalacia patellae. The management of this condition typically involves targeted strengthening exercises, patellar taping techniques and careful load management to reduce symptoms and improve function (Crossley et al., 2016).

Screening for Red Flags

It is important to screen for red flags during assessment of knee pain (Table 10.2). These include possible fractures, malignant lesions, infections and ligamentous injuries, as recommended by NICE (2023a). Knee scenarios and red flags are listed in Table 10.4.

Assessment Approach

The assessment of knee pain should be comprehensive, involving a detailed history, thorough physical examination and appropriate functional tests to guide diagnosis and management.

Management Principles

Initial management should focus on conservative measures, with surgical intervention considered only when these approaches are unsuccessful (Hunter and Bierma-Zeinstra, 2022).

Associated Factors

Experiencing pain during downhill activities may suggest issues related to the loading of the knee joint. Furthermore, increased body weight can exacerbate the intensity of knee pain.

Table 10.4 Knee clinical scenarios: pattern recognition and red flags.

Clinical scenario	Key clinical tests/ observations	Likely diagnosis/ pattern	Red flags/ additional considerations
1. 28-year-old male football player, twisting injury during football, swelling, redness, cannot bear weight, knee gives way constantly and feels unstable, held in flexed posture	Large joint effusion Positive Lachman or anterior drawer ↓ Extension Instability on knee rotation	ACL tear ± meniscal injury	Suspect haemarthrosis Refer to physiotherapy MRI referral via secondary referral if ongoing instability Rehab or ACL reconstruction depending on function and quality of life
2. 58-year-old male, sudden posterior knee swelling, redness, feeling unwell, tired, post chest infection for the past month	Swelling behind knee (Baker's cyst) Warmth, systemic symptoms – fever/chills/ malaise Reduced ROM, tenderness	Infection or inflammatory arthritis, e.g. septic arthritis or reactive arthritis	Red flag: systemic symptoms Urgent referral (emergency) Bloods: ESR, CRP, joint aspiration Rule out septic joint

(Continued)

Table 10.4 *(Continued)*

Clinical scenario	Key clinical tests/ observations	Likely diagnosis/ pattern	Red flags/ additional considerations
3. 38-year-old female, runner, pain with uphill running and kickboxing, desk-based work, systemically well	Anterior knee pain Pain ↑ with stairs, loading Patellofemoral joint tenderness	Patellofemoral pain syndrome (PFPS)/overuse tendinopathy	Conservative management Modify aggravating activity Strengthening programme – quads, glutes Physiotherapy referral for restoring function
4. 65-year-old female, knee bent and waddling gait, chronic pain worsening for the past 4–5 years, failed steroid injections (two in the past in two years), diabetes type II, overweight	Valgus/varus deformity ↓ ROM Crepitus X-ray: osteoarthritic changes	Advanced osteoarthritis with deformity	Consider joint replacement referral if quality of life is poor Screen for mobility aids, falls risk Physiotherapy referral for strengthening for lower limbs

Abbreviations: ACL, anterior cruciate ligament; CRP, C-reactive protein; ESR, erythrocyte sedimentation rate; ROM, range of motion.

CHAPTER 11

The Foot and Ankle

Introduction

The foot and ankle provide support, stability and propulsion during movement. They are prone to trauma, overuse injuries, degenerative conditions and systemic diseases. Foot and ankle pain may arise from musculoskeletal, neurological, inflammatory, vascular or systemic causes, requiring a thorough assessment (Standring, 2021). Common conditions seen in primary care affecting foot and ankle are listed in Table 11.1, red flags to be vigilant for in Table 11.2 and special tests for ankle assessments in Table 11.3.

Functions and Clinical Significance of the Foot and Ankle

The foot and ankle play a crucial role in providing support, maintaining balance and stability, and enabling propulsion during movement. Given their fundamental function in weight bearing and locomotion, these structures are particularly susceptible to a variety of problems. Trauma, overuse injuries, degenerative conditions, systemic diseases and inflammatory conditions can all adversely affect the foot and ankle.

Pain in this region may stem from a range of causes, including musculoskeletal, neurological, inflammatory, vascular or systemic origins. Consequently, it is essential to undertake a comprehensive assessment to accurately identify the underlying cause of foot and ankle pain (Standring, 2021).

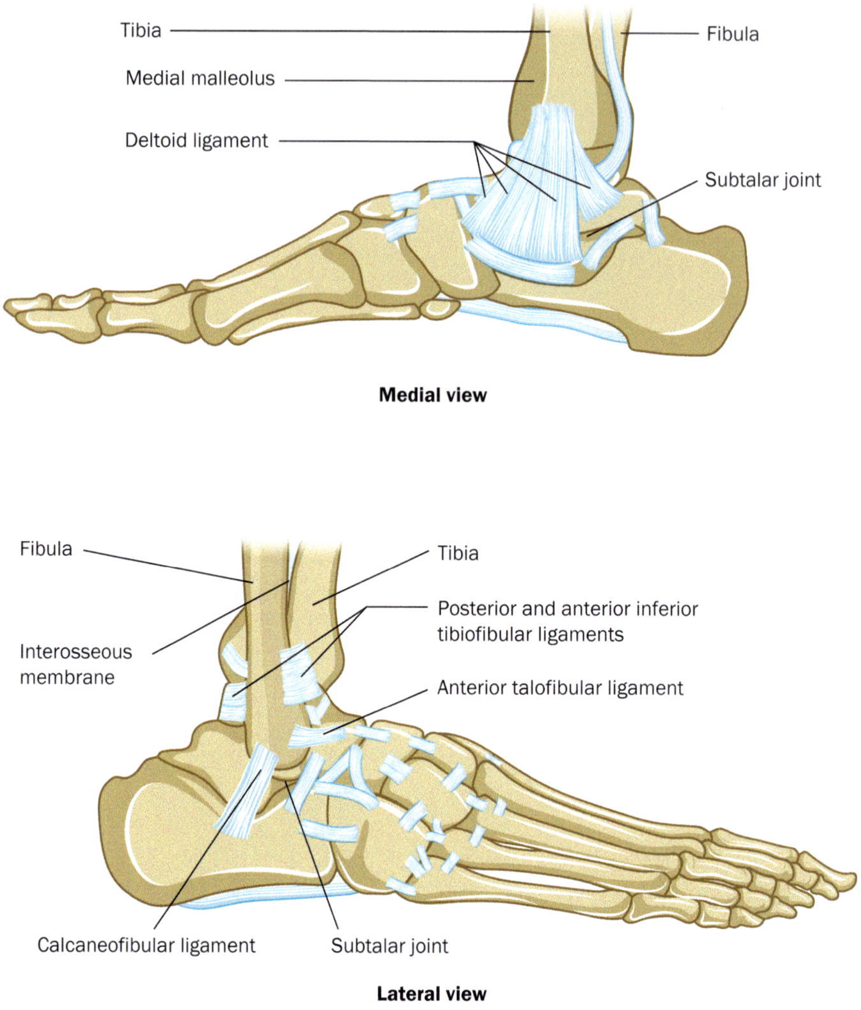

Figure 11.1 Foot and ankle anatomy.

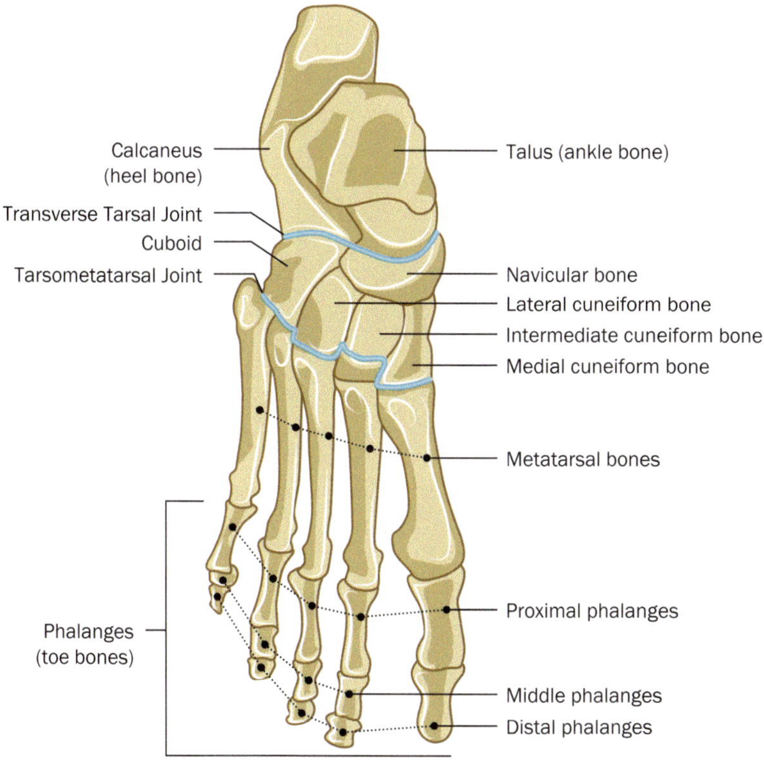

Figure 11.1 *(Continued)*

Anatomy Overview

The foot and ankle complex consists of the following aspects (Figure 11.1).

- **Bones** – Tibia, fibula, talus, calcaneus, tarsals, metatarsals, phalanges.
- **Joints** – Talocrural (ankle), subtalar, midfoot, metatarsophalangeal (MTP).
- **Ligaments** – Anterior talofibular ligament (ATFL), calcaneofibular ligament (CFL), deltoid ligament, plantar fascia.
- **Muscles and tendons** – Gastrocnemius, soleus, tibialis posterior, peroneal tendons.
- **Neurovascular supply** – Tibial nerve, peroneal nerve; posterior tibial artery (Standring, 2021).

Table 11.1 Common foot and ankle conditions.

Condition	Cause	Symptoms	Investigations	Management
Ankle sprain (ATFL/CFL injury)	Inversion injury Twisted ankle	Lateral ankle pain, swelling, instability, difficulty weight bearing, bruising	Clinical diagnosis X-ray to rule out fracture	PEACE and LOVE: **P**rotect **E**levate **A**void anti-inflammatories **C**ompression **E**ducation **L**oad **O**ptimism **V**ascularisation **E**xercise Physiotherapy referral Bracing/support and activity modification and functional rehab (Dubois and Esculier 2020)
Achilles tendinopathy	Overuse, repetitive strain, inflammatory, sports injury, degenerative tendon Bilateral with inflammatory conditions – axial spondyloarthropathy, psoriatic arthropathy	Posterior heel pain and stiffness, especially in the morning, with tendon tenderness and swelling	Clinical diagnosis Ultrasound if rupture is suspected	Taping, support, physiotherapy referral, functional rehab, activity modification, shockwave therapy if loading is not improving symptoms (Silbernagel et al., 2020)

Plantar fasciitis	Overuse, standing job, inflammatory, degenerative Overweight Inflammatory conditions – axial spondyloarthropathy, psoriatic arthropathy	Morning heel pain, especially with initial steps	Windlass test – With the patient supine, passively dorsiflex the ankle and toes If symptoms worsen, perform ultrasound	Advise loading (calf raises), stretching, orthotics, shockwave therapy, functional rehab, activity modification (Rasenberg et al., 2018)
Morton's neuroma	Compression of interdigital nerve	Forefoot pain, burning, worse with tight shoes/ heels Painful feeling of stone stuck in the shoe while walking	Mulder's click – When the examiner squeezes the toes at the metatarsophalangeal joint while the patient is lying supine, a positive test is indicated by the production of both pain and a clicking sensation Ultrasound via secondary care referral for injection/ intervention	Footwear modification, toe stretches, metatarsal pads, corticosteroid injection – under ultrasound guidance via secondary care referral (Mahadevan et al., 2015)
Tarsal tunnel syndrome	Tibial nerve compression at foot	Medial ankle pain, tingling in sole, age related, overuse, footwear issues	Tinel's sign at foot – Tapping on medial ankle joint reproduces paraesthesia, confirming tarsal tunnel syndrome Nerve conduction studies if symptoms worsen or for injection/intervention	Foot and ankle stretch, neural mobilisation via physiotherapy referral, activity modification, footwear change, surgical decompression if symptoms worsen (McSweeney and Cichero 2015)

Table 11.2 Red flags and emergency referral criteria for foot and ankle disorders.

Red flag	Potential serious condition	Immediate action
Acute pain and inability to bear weight after trauma/injury	Fracture of foot and ankle bones/joints Classification of this is explained in Table 11.4 Lisfranc injury – midfoot injury, fracture dislocation	Urgent X-ray, orthopaedic referral (Court-Brown et al., 2015)
Sudden-onset severe calf pain and tenderness + swelling + redness, breathlessness, inflammation Risk factors – Cardiovascular history, post-surgery, infection, cancer history, prolonged sitting, e.g. long-haul flight Pregnancy, obesity, oral contraceptives containing oestrogen	Deep vein thrombosis (DVT)	Refer to emergency Urgent Doppler ultrasound and D-dimer blood test Anticoagulation therapy for confirmed DVT (Kearon et al., 2019)
Progressive foot pain + unremitting night pain, unexplained weight loss >5% body weight in the past 6–12 months, fever, feeling unwell, fatigue, lump, unusual swelling without trauma, history of cancer	Bone tumour (osteosarcoma, metastases)	Urgent imaging via urgent suspected cancer pathway (Rosenberg et al., 2020)
Foot ulcer + peripheral neuropathy Secondary to diabetes, vasculitis Thyroid/liver/kidney issues Infections	Diabetic foot infection, osteomyelitis	Urgent vascular and podiatry referral (Armstrong et al., 2017)
Severe heel pain with systemic symptoms – fever/chills, difficulty weight bearing, feeling unwell, swelling, tenderness, inflammation	Septic arthritis, calcaneal osteomyelitis	Emergency referral for joint aspiration, IV antibiotics (Mathews et al., 2010)

Abbreviation: IV, intravenous.

Foot and Ankle Assessment Protocol

History Taking

- **Site of pain** – Heel (plantar fasciitis, Achilles), medial (tarsal tunnel), forefoot (neuroma).
- **Onset** – Acute (trauma) versus chronic (overuse, systemic).
- **Character** – Sharp, dull, burning, neuropathic.
- **Aggravating and relieving factors** – Activity, footwear, rest.
- **Systemic symptoms** – Fever, night pain, weight loss (Finucane et al., 2020).

Physical Examination

- **Observation** – Swelling, redness, bruising, inflammation, deformity, calluses, ulceration, anatomical variations.
- **Palpation** – Tenderness (Achilles, plantar fascia, MTP joints).
- **Range of motion (ROM)** – Dorsiflexion, plantarflexion, inversion, eversion; check forefoot and hindfoot.
- **Neurological examination** – Reflexes, dermatomes, myotomes (Magee, 2021)

Table 11.3 Special tests for foot and ankle conditions.

Test	Condition	Positive finding
Thompson test	Achilles tendon rupture	Plantarflexion observed following calf compression with the patient in a prone position indicates an intact Achilles tendon. Absence of movement suggests a rupture of the tendon (Silbernagel et al., 2020)
Windlass test	Plantar fasciitis	Pain with passive toe dorsiflexion suggests plantar fasciopathy (Rasenberg et al., 2018)
Mulder's click test	Morton's neuroma	Clicking sensation and pain with metatarsal squeeze (Mahadevan et al., 2015)
Tinel's sign	Tarsal tunnel syndrome	Tingling reproduced by tapping on medial ankle joint confirms nerve entrapment (McSweeney and Cichero 2015)
Ottawa Ankle Rules explained in detail below (Table 11.4)	Fracture screening	Pain with palpation over malleoli or inability to bear weight (Court-Brown et al., 2015)

Table 11.4 Ottawa ankle rules (Bessen et al., 2009).

Area	Criteria for X-ray	Clinical findings
Ankle X-ray required	Pain in the malleolar zone AND *at least one* of the following:	Palpable pain along the distal 6 cm of the fibula
	Bone tenderness at the posterior edge or tip of the lateral malleolus	Palpable pain along the distal 6 cm of the tibia
	Bone tenderness at the posterior edge or tip of the medial malleolus	Unable to take 4 steps immediately after injury and in the ED
	Inability to weight bear	
Foot X-ray required	Pain in the mid-foot zone AND *at least one* of the following:	Pain on palpation of the tuberosity
	Bone tenderness at the base of the 5th metatarsal	Pain on palpation of the navicular bone
	Bone tenderness at the navicular	Unable to take 4 steps immediately after injury and in the ED
	Inability to weight bear	
Exclusions – not applicable if	Under 18 years	Skeletally immature
	Intoxicated/unreliable history	Impaired assessment
	Multiple injuries	Distracting pain
	Reduced sensation	Neurological compromise
	Gross swelling preventing palpation	Limits clinical accuracy

Management Strategies for Foot and Ankle Conditions

Conservative Management

- **Education and activity modification** – Footwear advice, load management, education, reassurance, psychological support.
- **Physiotherapy referral** – Strengthening, stretching, balance and stability exercises.
- **Pain relief** – NSAIDs, paracetamol, orthotics, taping, ankle support (Silbernagel et al., 2020).

Interventional Management (When Conservative Treatment Fails)

- **Corticosteroid injections** – For Morton's neuroma and ankle joint OA.
- **Surgical referral.**

- **For chronic Achilles rupture** (tendon repair).
- **For severe hallux valgus** (bunionectomy).
- **For Lisfranc injuries** (internal fixation) (Mahadevan et al., 2015).

Key Takeaways

The foot and ankle are particularly susceptible to a range of injuries and degenerative changes, often arising from trauma or repetitive overuse. These structures commonly present with conditions such as ankle sprains, Achilles tendinopathy, plantar fasciitis and Morton's neuroma (Dubois and Esculier 2020).

Screening and Assessment

It is essential to remain vigilant for red flags during evaluation, including the possibility of fractures, malignancy, deep vein thrombosis (DVT) and infections (NICE, 2023b) (Table 11.5). A thorough and structured assessment is necessary and should encompass a detailed history, physical examination and relevant special tests (Magee, 2021).

Management Approach

Treatment strategies must be individualised, considering both the severity and underlying cause of the symptoms (Silbernagel et al., 2020).

Inflammatory Arthritis Considerations

For cases where dactylitis is present, particularly with axial or psoriatic inflammatory arthritis, further details are available in Chapter 12. Additionally, bilateral Achilles tendonitis and plantar fasciitis are more suggestive of underlying inflammatory arthritis and should prompt referral to rheumatology and physiotherapy for a comprehensive approach.

Table 11.5 Foot and ankle clinical scenarios: pattern recognition and red flags.

Clinical scenario	Key clinical tests/observations	Likely diagnosis/pattern	Red flags/additional considerations
1. 78-year-old male, lives alone, on chemotherapy for prostate cancer, long history of hypertension, presents with pitting oedema, tender swollen calf, warm calf and struggling to bear weight	Pitting oedema Calf tenderness ↑ Risk: malignancy + immobility No trauma history	Deep vein thrombosis (DVT)	Urgent emergency referral for Doppler Ultrasound to rule out DVT and D-dimer blood test Red flag: cancer + hypertension and calf tenderness + swelling

(*Continued*)

Table 11.5 (*Continued*)

Clinical scenario	Key clinical tests/ observations	Likely diagnosis/ pattern	Red flags/additional considerations
2. 16-year-old female netball player, limping after the game, severe heel pain for few days, swelling on the ankle, no trauma	Tenderness posterior ankle Pain ↑ with walking/standing/ stairs activity Growth spurt history	Sever's disease (calcaneal apophysitis)	Common in active teenagers Progressive loading rehab advice Physiotherapy referral if symptoms worsen
3. 46-year-old female, retail worker, daily usage of heels, reported worsening pain in forefoot, worse with walking, burning pain and paraesthesia reported with walking	Pain between 2nd and 4th toes Positive Mulder's click Worse in tight shoes Localised forefoot tenderness	Morton's neuroma	Common in women, heel wearers Orthotics – metatarsal pads Footwear modification Ultrasound-guided steroid injection if symptoms persist
4. 52-year-old male, teacher, pain in the morning, worsens with walking, unable to bear weight for long time after day's work	Plantar heel pain Windlass test positive Morning pain pattern Tight fascia	Plantar fasciopathy	Classic presentation Responds to stretches, orthotics Heel support/night splints may help if symptoms worsen

CHAPTER 12

Rheumatology

Introduction

The specialty of rheumatology includes over 200 rheumatic and musculoskeletal diseases (RMDs) which encompass a spectrum of degenerative, autoinflammatory and autoimmune conditions predominantly affecting the joints (Maini et al., 2020). 'Autoinflammatory' diseases and 'autoimmune' diseases represent two ends of this spectrum and include conditions such as rheumatoid arthritis (RA), polymyalgia rheumatica (PMR), systemic lupus erythematosus (SLE) and spondyloarthritis (SpA) (Szekanecz et al., 2021).

Rheumatic and musculoskeletal diseases range from relatively common to very rare and can be challenging to identify in primary care. Often, the non-specific nature of symptoms, or overlapping features, add to the diagnostic challenge outside specialist settings and contribute to delayed diagnosis (Ingram et al., 2025; Siddle et al., 2023).

Rheumatic and musculoskeletal diseases have variable prevalence, particularly with regard to axial SpA (Bohn et al., 2018), whereas in RA the condition affects ~1–2% of the population globally (Almutairi et al., 2021), and psoriatic arthritis (PsA) affects ~0.3–1% of the population (Gladman et al., 2005). It is important for primary care clinicians to be aware of such RMDs, their clinical presentation, relevant investigation and management. Prompt diagnosis of RMDs is crucial to optimise long-term patient outcomes and prevent the degree of physical and mental disability that ensues because of delayed diagnosis.

This chapter outlines the 'essentials' for primary care colleagues, empowering them to recognise RMDs early, raise their clinical 'index of suspicion' and enable timely and appropriate referrals through to rheumatology specialist teams. Common conditions and red flags are listed in Table 12.1 and Table 12.2.

Examination of Rheumatic and Musculoskeletal Diseases

Following a thorough subjective consultation, the core principles of a comprehensive objective musculoskeletal (MSK) assessment in primary care include a detailed examination of the MSK system. For RMDs, this includes observation, palpation, range of motion (ROM) and strength testing (Gross et al., 2015).

The MSK assessment should focus on the joints affected by the RMD in question and include a full neurological examination of upper and lower limbs, gait analysis and a battery of upper motor neuron tests.

Observation

- Assess posture, gait, alignment, joint deformity, muscle wasting and visual signs of joint swelling.
- Look for asymmetry and joint deformity (Stone et al., 2009).

Palpation

Check for joint-line tenderness and muscle tension (Stone et al., 2009).

Range of Motion Testing

- Assess joint movement such as flexion, extension, rotation, side flexion of the cervical spine.
- Painful and/or limited movements suggest joint dysfunction or soft tissue injury (Clarkson, 2020).

Neurological Examination

- Dermatomes – Sensory testing.
- Myotomes – Motor strength assessment.
- Upper and/or lower limb reflexes (Gross et al., 2015).

Though rarely undertaken in a primary care setting, the MSK examination can be expanded further for RMDs, tailored to specific diseases, by utilising such measures as the 28-joint Diseases Activity Score (DAS-28) in RA (Salaffi et al., 2021) or the Bath Ankylosing Spondylitis Metrology Index (BASMI), for axial spondyloarthritis, an internationally used composite index of spinal mobility used in research and clinical practice for those with SpA (Jenkinson et al., 1994). Conditions, red flags and scenarios are listed in Table 12.2.

Table 12.1 Summary of rheumatological conditions.

Condition	Cause	Symptoms	Investigations	Management
Rheumatoid arthritis (RA)	Autoimmune and autoinflammatory synovitis; genetic and environmental triggers	Bilateral small joint pain/swelling (hands, wrists, feet), stiffness, fatigue, possible cervical spine involvement	Serology (RF, anti-CCP), inflammatory markers, X-rays, 2010 ACR/EULAR classification criteria	Early referral: DMARDs (csDMARDs, bDMARDs), symptom control, treat-to-target strategy (Aletaha and Smolen, 2018; Allen et al., 2018; Bullock et al., 2018; Hammam et al., 2024; Kay and Upchurch, 2012; NICE, 2018)
Polymyalgia rheumatica (PMR)	Unknown; age >50, more common in women	Acute-onset bilateral shoulder and hip girdle pain/stiffness, fatigue, low-grade fever	Diagnosis of exclusion; inflammatory markers (ESR, CRP); NICE PMR guidance	Oral corticosteroids (12.5–25 mg prednisolone); slow tapering; monitor for relapse or GCA (Dejaco et al., 2015; Donskov et al., 2023; Espígol-Frigolé et al., 2023; Hysa et al., 2025; Ramon et al., 2022)
Gout	Monosodium urate crystal deposition, often due to hyperuricaemia	Acute monoarthritis (1st MTPJ common), pain, redness, swelling, rapid onset	Joint aspiration + polarised light microscopy, serum uric acid (may be normal in flare)	NSAIDs, colchicine, corticosteroids; urate-lowering therapy (ULT); lifestyle modification (Abhishek et al., 2017; Hui et al., 2017; NICE, 2022b; Roddy et al., 2024; Weaver et al., 2021)

(Continued)

Table 12.1 *(Continued)*

Condition	Cause	Symptoms	Investigations	Management
Pseudogout	Calcium pyrophosphate crystal deposition (CPPD)	Acute arthritis-like gout; commonly knees, wrists	Joint aspiration, X-rays (chondrocalcinosis)	NSAIDs, colchicine, corticosteroids (as for gout) (Borghi et al., 2020; Vambe et al., 2024)
Osteoporosis	Low bone mineral density due to ageing, hormonal factors, glucocorticoid use, RMDs	Often asymptomatic until fracture; common fracture sites include vertebrae, hip, wrist	DEXA scan, FRAX score	Vitamin D and calcium, bisphosphonates, lifestyle advice, exercise, fall prevention (Brooke-Wavell et al., 2022; Buttgereit et al., 2024; Cortet et al., 2024; Fuggle et al., 2024; Schini et al., 2024; Willers et al., 2022)
Axial spondyloarthritis (AxSpA)	Chronic inflammatory arthritis linked to HLA-B27	Inflammatory back pain, morning stiffness, alternating buttock pain, kyphosis in severe cases	MRI (sacroiliitis, enthesitis), X-ray for structural changes	NSAIDs, physiotherapy, exercise, biologics if needed (anti-TNF, IL-17 inhibitors) (Elshahawy et al., 2022; Ingram et al., 2025; Jenkinson et al., 1994; Ramiro et al., 2023; Van Der Heijde et al., 2017)
Psoriatic arthritis (PsA)	Inflammatory arthritis associated with psoriasis	Peripheral arthritis, dactylitis, enthesitis, nail changes, axial involvement	Clinical assessment, imaging, inflammatory markers	NSAIDs, csDMARDs, bDMARDs (TNF, IL inhibitors), tailored therapy per EULAR guidelines (Gladman et al., 2005; Gossec et al., 2020; Poddubnyy et al., 2021; Tillett et al., 2021; Zabotti et al., 2020)

Systemic lupus erythematosus (SLE)	Chronic autoimmune condition affecting multiple organs	Fatigue, rash, arthritis, nephritis, photosensitivity, oral ulcers, fever	ANA, dsDNA, complement levels, urinalysis, ACR/EULAR criteria	Immunosuppressants (steroids, hydroxychloroquine, azathioprine), regular monitoring (Ameer et al., 2022; Aringer et al., 2019; Fanouriakis et al., 2021; Siegel and Sammaritano, 2024)
Fibromyalgia syndrome (FMS)	Unknown; central sensitisation; often coexists with RMDs	Widespread pain, fatigue, sleep disturbance, cognitive dysfunction	Clinical diagnosis (WPI/SSS); exclude other causes	Education, graded exercise, CBT, duloxetine, amitriptyline; avoid NSAIDs (Berwick et al., 2022; Falasinnu et al., 2022; Jones et al., 2024; Macfarlane et al., 2017; Srinivasan et al., 2019)

Abbreviations: ANA, antinuclear antibody; CBT, cognitive behavioural therapy; CCP, cyclic citrullinated peptide; CRP, C-reactive protein; DEXA, dual-energy X-ray absorptiometry; DMARD, disease-modifying antirheumatic drug; ESR, erythrocyte sedimentation rate; FRAX, fracture risk assessment tool; GCA, giant cell arteritis; IL, interleukin; MTPJ, metatarsophalangeal joint; MRI, magnetic resonance imaging; NSAID, non-steroidal anti-inflammatory drug; RF, rheumatoid factor; SSS, symptom severity scale; TNF, tumour necrosis factor; WPI, widespread pain index.

Key Takeaways

- Tenosynovitis refers to inflammation of the synovial membrane surrounding tendons. It is a critical consideration for primary care practitioners and is increasingly recognised as an early indicator of RMDs such as rheumatoid arthritis (Niemantsverdriet and Van Der Helm-van Mil, 2018).
- Approximately 15–21% of patients with PMR exhibit associated giant cell arteritis (GCA), which may result in serious vascular complications (Ramon et al., 2022). Furthermore, 40–60% of individuals diagnosed with GCA also report symptoms consistent with PMR (Hysa et al., 2025).
- The prevalence of gout is between two and six times higher in males compared to females (Weaver et al., 2021).
- Nocturnal wakening during the latter half of the night due to back pain, in addition to alternating buttock pain, are characteristic features indicative of inflammatory back pain in spondyloarthritis (Elshahawy et al., 2022).
- Psoriatic arthritis predominantly develops in patients already diagnosed with cutaneous psoriasis; however, in approximately 15% of cases, psoriasis arises following the onset of arthritis or arthralgia (Zabotti et al., 2020).
- Clinicians should inquire about potential connective tissue disease manifestations, including hair loss or thinning, oral and nasal ulcers, dermatological rashes and Raynaud's phenomenon (Alves and Goncalo, 2019).
- Fibromyalgia syndrome is a prevalent and multifaceted condition characterised by persistent, widespread pain and can be reliably diagnosed in primary care or other non-specialist settings by qualified medical professionals (Berwick et al., 2022).
- Connective tissue diseases (CTDs) are infrequent disorders distinguished by a wide range of systemic and cutaneous presentations, often demonstrating variable and non-specific clinical features (Aringer et al., 2019; Asif et al., 2023; Ferrara et al., 2023).

Table 12.2 Rheumatology clinical scenarios: pattern recognition and red flags.

Clinical scenario	Key clinical tests/ observations	Likely diagnosis/ pattern	Red flags/ additional considerations
1. 32-year-old female, desk-based worker, reported long-standing back pain, worse with sitting, better with yoga/swimming, now has Achilles tendinitis and redness in eyes	Inflammatory back pain (AM stiffness >30 min) Enthesitis (Achilles) Inflammation of iris, changes may hint at uveitis Responds to exercise, not rest	Axial spondyloarthritis (AxSpA)	MRI whole spine Rheumatology referral Screen for psoriasis, uveitis, inflammatory bowel disease

Clinical scenario	Key clinical tests/ observations	Likely diagnosis/ pattern	Red flags/ additional considerations
2. 75-year-old male, sudden swelling in both hands, struggling to shave and support wife with daily chores, early morning stiffness for 40 mins for the past few weeks, tired, feeling weak in his hands	Symmetrical small joint swelling ↓ Grip strength Prolonged AM stiffness Synovitis on palpation	Rheumatoid arthritis (RA)	Classic in older adults Serology: RF, anti-CCP Urgent rheumatology referral
3. 56-year-old female, reported pain in both shoulder + hip since past 1.5 months, increasing fatigue, struggling to rise from chair (classic chair sign), tired	Bilateral proximal stiffness Morning pain >45 min ↑ ESR/CRP Rapid response to low-dose steroids	Polymyalgia rheumatica (PMR)	Age >50, rapid onset Rule out GCA if headache/vision change and jaw tenderness Long tapering course of prednisolone in primary care
4. 43-year-old female, gradual worsening facial rash, worsened skin issues when exposed to sun, joint pain and aches, feels tired and weak	Malar ('butterfly') rash Polyarthralgia Photosensitivity Systemic fatigue Mouth ulcers	Systemic lupus erythematosus (SLE)	Blood tests – ANA, dsDNA, complement levels Multisystem monitoring (skin, kidneys, CNS) Rheumatology referral essential

Abbreviations: ANA, antinuclear antibody; CCP, cyclic citrullinated peptide; CNS, central nervous system; CRP, C-reactive protein; ESR, erythrocyte sedimentation rate; GCA, giant cell arteritis; MRI, magnetic resonance imaging; RF, rheumatoid factor.

CHAPTER 13

Musculoskeletal Guidelines and Pathways

Musculoskeletal Assessment and Management

Musculoskeletal (MSK) assessment and management in contemporary clinical practice are underpinned by a thorough evidence base, supported by national guidelines and emerging research (Table 13.1). Effective MSK care requires a structured approach to clinical reasoning that integrates comprehensive patient assessment, accurate diagnosis, appropriate referral pathways and personalised management strategies. Current guidance emphasises the importance of integrating research evidence with clinical expertise to optimise outcomes, reduce variation in care and promote high-value practice across primary and secondary care settings (NICE, 2021a).

A systematic and hypothesis-driven assessment is central to identifying the nature and severity of MSK presentations, distinguishing between benign mechanical conditions and those requiring urgent medical or surgical intervention. Contemporary models advocate for the use of validated screening tools, functional assessment and psychosocial evaluation to inform diagnostic decision making and management planning (Oliveira et al., 2021). Such approaches recognise the multifactorial nature of MSK conditions and the necessity of tailoring interventions to the individual patient.

Person-centred Care

Person-centred care is a fundamental component of modern MSK practice. It requires clinicians to incorporate the patient's ideas, concerns, expectations, values and lived experiences into all stages of assessment and management. This approach is strongly associated with improved therapeutic engagement, enhanced adherence to treatment plans and greater patient satisfaction (Elwyn et al., 2020). Within MSK settings, shared decision making has been shown to reduce unnecessary imaging, inappropriate referrals and unwarranted variation in treatment, thereby supporting both clinical and economic efficiency (NICE, 2021a).

Person-centred practice extends beyond the provision of information; it entails collaborative goal setting, transparent communication about prognosis and active discussion of treatment preferences. Evidence suggests that when patients feel involved in decisions about their care, outcomes including pain, function and psychological well-being are significantly improved (Oliveira et al., 2021).

Safety and Prognosis

Ensuring patient safety is a core priority in MSK management. Screening for red flags – clinical indicators of potentially serious pathology such as malignancy, fracture, spinal infection or cauda equina syndrome – remains an essential component of assessment. Table 13.2 captures red flags in all regions.

However, contemporary evidence highlights the limited specificity of individual red flags, underscoring the need for careful interpretation within the broader clinical context rather than reliance on isolated findings (Downie et al., 2013; Karran et al., 2022).

Safety netting has emerged as a critical strategy for addressing diagnostic uncertainty. It involves providing patients with clear guidance on red flag symptoms, expected trajectories of recovery and instructions on when to revisit or escalate care. Robust safety netting has been shown to reduce diagnostic delay, facilitate timely intervention in cases of deterioration and improve patient confidence in self-management (Albury et al., 2022).

Prognosis in MSK conditions is influenced by a complex interplay of biological, psychological and social factors. Evidence-based management emphasises early identification of modifiable risk factors, ongoing monitoring of symptom progression and timely referral to specialist services when required. Timely and appropriate imaging is recommended for musculoskeletal conditions within the limitations of primary care. Table 13.3 summarises the necessary investigations for all the regions. These principles enhance clinical safety, support optimal long-term outcomes and align care delivery with high-quality MSK practice standards (Finucane et al., 2020; NICE, 2024a).

A critical component of MSK assessment in primary care practice is recognising when a patient's symptoms may be influenced or even caused by medications rather than underlying MSK pathology. Several commonly prescribed drugs can produce side-effects that closely resemble MSK conditions, leading to misdiagnosis, unnecessary imaging or inappropriate referral if not identified early.

Statins, for example, are widely prescribed for cardiovascular risk reduction, yet are well known to cause myalgia and proximal muscle weakness that may mimic polymyalgia rheumatica, cervical/lumbar radiculopathy or generalised inflammatory conditions (NICE, 2024b). Systemic corticosteroids, although used therapeutically in many inflammatory disorders, can paradoxically contribute to proximal myopathy and significantly increase osteoporosis and fragility fracture risk when used long term (NICE, 2022b; NICE, 2024b). Similarly, fluoroquinolone antibiotics carry a recognised MHRA warning for tendon injury and rupture, particularly affecting the Achilles tendon, and should be considered in any new-onset tendon pain especially in older adults or those also taking steroids (MHRA, 2019).

Medicines increasingly used in chronic pain management such as opioids and gabapentinoids also complicate MSK assessment. Opioids may worsen functional impairment through sedation, falls risk, constipation-related pelvic/back pain and opioid-induced hyperalgesia, and are therefore not recommended for chronic primary pain (NICE, 2020). Gabapentinoids can cause dizziness, ataxia and gait disturbance, sometimes mimicking radiculopathy or myelopathy, and contribute significantly to falls risk (NICE, 2020). Antidepressants such as SSRIs, SNRIs and TCAs, although beneficial in certain pain phenotypes, may also cause orthostatic hypotension and sedation, requiring caution in frail or older adults (NICE, 2020).

In addition, some medications exert indirect MSK effects. Long-term proton pump inhibitors (PPIs) can reduce calcium and magnesium absorption and are associated with increased fracture risk (NICE, 2024b), while antihypertensives may cause dizziness or postural hypotension that affects balance, confidence and physical activity participation (NICE, 2024b).

Understanding these medication-related effects allows clinicians to differentiate true MSK pathology from drug-induced symptoms, optimise prescribing, minimise harm and support more accurate diagnosis. For many patients with persistent, vague or widespread MSK symptoms, a careful medication review can be just as important as physical examination in forming an accurate clinical picture (Table 13.4).

Table 13.1 MSK guidelines and pharmacology.

Area	Condition/topic	NICE guideline/CKS	Core messages (high level)
Spine	Low back pain ± sciatica	NICE (2016a)	Clinical diagnosis; avoid routine imaging; exercise and activity as first line; manual therapy only as part of a package; consider psychological therapies; MRI only if it will change management or for progressive neurological deficit/ surgical planning (NICE, 2016a)

(Continued)

Table 13.1 (*Continued*)

Area	**Condition/topic**	**NICE guideline/CKS**	**Core messages (high level)**
Spine	Neck/thoracic pain	NICE (2016a) NICE (2024b) NICE (2024c) NICE (2024d)	Screen for red flags; manage most cases conservatively with advice and exercise; imaging only if red flags or trauma are suspected (NICE, 2024c)
Osteoarthritis	Osteoarthritis (hip, knee, hand)	NICE (2022a)	Clinical diagnosis; exercise and weight loss core; topical NSAIDs first line; oral NSAIDs + PPI when needed; intra-articular steroid injections for flares; avoid PRP or hyaluronic acid; surgery based on symptoms and function, not age/BMI (NICE, 2022a)
Pain	Chronic primary pain	NICE (2020)	Quality-of-life focus; exercise; CBT-type interventions; acupuncture; avoid opioids, gabapentinoids, NSAIDs, paracetamol, benzodiazepines; consider antidepressants (NICE, 2020)
Inflammatory	Rheumatoid arthritis	NICE (2018)	Urgent referral within three working days; early DMARD therapy; treat-to-target; monitor for comorbidity and drug toxicity (NICE, 2018)
Inflammatory	Axial/peripheral spondyloarthritis	NICE (2017)	Consider in <45-year inflammatory back pain; MRI preferred; NSAIDs first line; biologics in specialist care (NICE, 2017)
Crystal	Gout	NICE (2022b)	NSAIDs/colchicine/oral steroids for acute flare; early urate-lowering therapy ULT; treat-to-target serum urate (NICE, 2022b)
Systemic	PMR and GCA	NICE (2024q) NICE (2024r)	PMR: shoulder/hip girdle stiffness + raised ESR/CRP; rapid steroid response. GCA: headache/jaw claudication/visual disturbance → same-day steroids and urgent referral (NICE, 2024q; NICE, 2024r)

Area	Condition/topic	NICE guideline/CKS	Core messages (high level)
Soft tissue (upper limb)	RCRSP, frozen shoulder, tennis/golfer's elbow, De Quervain's, trigger finger	NICE (2024b) NICE (2024j) NICE (2024k) NICE (2024l) NICE (2024m)	Clinical diagnosis; exercise and load management first line; injections in select cases; imaging only when management changes (NICE, 2024b; NICE, 2024k; NICE, 2024j; NICE, 2024l; NICE, 2024m)
Soft tissue (lower limb)	GTPS, plantar fasciitis, Achilles tendinopathy, PF pain	NICE (2024e) NICE (2024f) NICE (2024g) NICE (2024h) NICE (2024i)	Exercise and load modification; eccentric training where appropriate; avoid steroid injections into Achilles (NICE, 2024e; NICE, 2024f; NICE, 2024g; NICE, 2024h; NICE, 2024e; NICE, 2024i)
Trauma	Non-complex fractures	NICE (2016b)	Ottawa Rules for imaging; immobilise and support early movement (NICE, 2016b)
Trauma	Complex fractures/major trauma	NICE (2016c) NICE (2016d)	Specialist management; early stabilisation; trauma networks (NICE, 2016c; NICE, 2016d)
Bone health	Osteoporosis	NICE (2024o)	Risk stratification with FRAX/Q-Fracture; DEXA scanning; bisphosphonates first line; falls prevention (NICE, 2024o)
System	Shared decision making	NICE (2021a)	'No decision about me, without me'; explain options, benefits, risks (NICE, 2021a)
System	MSK pathway/ GIRFT	NICE (2024)	Navigation hub for all MSK guidance; GIRFT emphasises reducing variation, avoiding unnecessary MRI/injections/ opioids and optimising referral (GIRFT, 2020a; NICE, 2024)

Abbreviations: BMI, body mass index; CBT, cognitive behavioural therapy; CRP, C-reactive protein; DEXA, dual-energy X-ray absorptiometry; DMARD, disease-modifying antirheumatic drug; ESR, erythrocyte sedimentation rate; GCA, giant cell arteritis; GIRFT, Get It Right First Time; GTPS, greater trochanteric pain syndrome; MRI, magnetic resonance imaging; MSK, musculoskeletal; NSAID, non-steroidal anti-inflammatory drug; PF, patellofemoral; PMR; polymyalgia rheumatica; PPI, protein pump inhibitor; PRP, platelet-rich plasma; RCRSP, rotator cuff-related shoulder pain; ULT, urate lowering therapy.

Table 13.2 Red flags in all regions.

Region	Red flag examples	Serious pathology	Action
Spine	Saddle anaesthesia, urinary retention/incontinence, bilateral sciatica	Cauda equina syndrome	Same-day emergency referral (NICE, 2016a)
Spine	Fever, night pain, IVDU, immunosuppression	Spinal infection	Urgent CT/MRI, labs (NICE, 2016a; NICE, 2024a)
Spine	Cancer history, unexplained weight loss	Malignancy	Suspected cancer pathway (NICE, 2015)
Upper limb	Hot swollen joint + fever	Septic arthritis	Same-day medical review (NICE, 2024a)
Lower limb	Calf swelling, SOB	DVT/PE	Urgent VTE pathway (NICE, 2023b)
Systemic	New headache, jaw claudication, visual loss	GCA	Immediate high-dose steroids + same-day referral (NICE, 2024r)
Multiple joints	Synovitis + >60-minute stiffness	Early RA	Urgent rheumatology referral (NICE, 2018)

Abbreviations: CT, computed tomography; DVT, deep vein thrombosis; GCA, giant cell arteritis; IVDU, intravenous drug use; MRI, magnetic resonance imaging; PE, pulmonary embolism; RA, rheumatoid arthritis; SOB, shortness of breath; VTE, venous thromboembolism.

Table 13.3 Imaging decisions in common MSK presentations.

Clinical area	When to image	Rationale
Non-specific LBP	**Do not routinely image**	Imaging does not improve outcomes (NICE, 2016a)
Sciatica	MRI via secondary care referral if progressive deficit or considering surgery	To confirm nerve root involvement (NICE, 2016a)
Knee pain	X-ray for suspected OA; MRI via secondary care referral for locking/giving way	MRI via secondary care referral only if management changes (NICE, 2024e)
Shoulder pain	Ultrasound/MRI via secondary care referral if traumatic tear suspected or considering surgery	Avoid routine imaging (NICE, 2024b)
Ankle/knee trauma	Ottawa Rules to determine X-ray	Reduce unnecessary imaging (NICE, 2016b)
Inflammatory arthritis	MRI/US via secondary care referral (specialist)	For synovitis/erosion assessment (NICE, 2017)
Suspected malignancy/infection	Urgent CT/MRI via secondary care referral	Based on red flag assessment (NICE, 2015)

Abbreviations: MRI, magnetic resonance imaging; OA, osteoarthritis; US, ultrasound.

Table 13.4 Medicines that mimic or worsen musculoskeletal symptoms.

Drug group	MSK-relevant effects	Clinical implication
Statins	Myalgia, proximal muscle pain/weakness	Can mimic PMR, cervical/lumbar radiculopathy or inflammatory conditions. Always consider statin-induced myopathy as a differential (NICE, 2024p)
Systemic corticosteroids	Proximal myopathy, osteoporosis, increased fracture risk	Prolonged use weakens bone and muscle, increasing fragility fracture risk and masking inflammatory conditions (NICE, 2024o)
Fluoroquinolone antibiotics	Tendinopathy and tendon rupture, especially Achilles	MHRA warns of severe tendon injury; avoid excessive loading and consider this in sudden tendon pain (MHRA Drug Safety Update, 2019)
Opioids	Sedation, constipation (may worsen pelvic/back pain), falls risk, opioid-induced hyperalgesia	Should *not* be used for chronic primary pain due to harm > benefit (NICE, 2020). High vigilance in frailty and fall-prone patients
Gabapentinoids	Sedation, dizziness, gait disturbance, peripheral oedema	Can mimic neurological conditions (myelopathy/radiculopathy) and contribute to falls; avoid initiation in chronic primary pain (NICE, 2020)
Antidepressants (TCAs, SSRIs, SNRIs)	Drowsiness, dizziness, postural hypotension	Important in balance disorders and frailty; although duloxetine/amitriptyline may help chronic primary pain (NICE, 2020)
PPIs	Reduced calcium/magnesium absorption, ↑ fracture risk	Long-term PPI use associated with increased fragility fracture risk, requiring consideration in bone health assessments (NICE, 2024o)
Antihypertensives	Dizziness, orthostatic hypotension	Contributes to balance problems, falls, and reduced exercise tolerance – especially relevant in MSK rehab (NICE, 2024s)

Abbreviations: PPI, proton pump inhibitor; SNRI, serotonin noradrenaline reuptake inhibitor; SSRI, selective serotonin reuptake inhibitor; TCA, tricyclic antidepressant.

The following tables present several generalised pathways that impact all regions: osteoarthritis guidelines (Figure 13.1), chronic primary pain pathway (Figure 13.2), early inflammatory pathway (Figure 13.3), soft tissue pathway (Figure 13.4) and suspected fracture/trauma pathway (Figure 13.5).

PATIENT WITH JOINT PAIN (KNEE/HIP/HAND, ≥45 YEARS)

History and examination:
- Activity-related pain?
- Morning stiffness <30 minutes?
- No major red flags?

⇩

Typical OA clinical features present?

⇩ YES ⇩

Diagnose OA clinically
NO routine imaging required

⇩ NO ⇩

Consider alternative diagnoses;
investigate or refer as appropriate

⇩

EXPLAIN DIAGNOSIS and OPTIONS
- Nature of OA
- Role of lifestyle and exercise
- Long-term outlook

⇩

CORE TREATMENTS FOR ALL:
- Exercise (strength + aerobic)
- Weight management (if overweight)
- Education, pacing, activity modification

⇩

SYMPTOM CONTROL:
1. Topical NSAIDs (knee/hand)
2. Oral NSAIDs + PPI if needed
3. Consider intra-articular steroid injections for flares or short-term relief

⇩

REVIEW FUNCTION, PAIN, QUALITY OF LIFE

⇩	⇩
Adequate function/ manageable pain	Persistent pain, marked functional limitation
Ongoing conservative management, self-management, monitoring	Consider referral for joint replacement if: significant impact on QoL AND conservative measures optimised. Age/BMI alone MUST NOT exclude surgery.

Figure 13.1 Osteoarthritis guidelines (NICE NG226 [NICE, 2022a]).

PATIENT WITH PAIN >3 MONTHS

Comprehensive assessment:
- Pain characteristics (location, pattern)
- Functional impact
- Mood, sleep, coping, beliefs
- Screen for red flags and specific pathology

⇩

CLEAR STRUCTURAL/DISEASE CAUSE?

⇩ YES

⇩

Follow relevant NICE guideline (OA, RA, gout fracture, etc.)

⇩ NO

⇩

Consider CHRONIC PRIMARY PAIN diagnosis

⇩

EXPLAIN CHRONIC PRIMARY PAIN:
- Pain as a condition in its own right
- Aim to improve function and QoL, not necessarily to remove all pain

⇩

OFFER NON-PHARMACOLOGICAL CARE:
- Supported exercise programme
- Psychological therapies (CBT-based)
- Multidisciplinary pain management
- Acupuncture (where available)

⇩

MEDICINES (CAUTIOUS):
- Consider antidepressants (e.g. amitriptyline, duloxetine) after shared decision making
- DO NOT initiate opioids, gabapentinoids, NSAIDs, paracetamol, benzodiazepines or corticosteroid injections for chronic primary pain

⇩

ONGOING REVIEW:
- Collaborative goal setting
- Monitor function, mood, sleep, participation
- De-prescribe ineffective/harmful medicines
- Reinforce self-management and pacing

Figure 13.2 Chronic primary pain pathway (NICE NG193 [NICE, 2020]).

PATIENT WITH JOINT OR BACK PAIN

⇩

History and examination:
- Small joint swelling?
- Prolonged morning stiffness (>60 min)?
- Back pain starting <45 years, improving with exercise?
- Systemic symptoms (fatigue, weight loss, fever)?
- Skin psoriasis, IBD, uveitis?

⇩

SIGNS OF INFLAMMATORY ARTHRITIS?
(RA type, SpA type, multi-joint synovitis)

⇩ YES

⇩

URGENT RHEUMATOLOGY REFERRAL (within ~3 working days) (NG65 [NICE, 2017], NG100 [NICE, 2018])

⇩

For older adults with:
- Bilateral shoulder/hip girdle pain
- Marked morning stiffness
- Raised ESR/CRP

→ SUSPECT PMR (CKS PMR)

⇩

CHECK FOR GCA SYMPTOMS:
- New headache
- Scalp tenderness
- Jaw claudication
- Visual disturbance

⇩ YES

⇩

Start HIGH-DOSE oral steroids IMMEDIATELY + same-day urgent referral (ophthalmology/medicine) (CKS GCA)

⇩ NO

⇩

Treat as PMR with standard-dose steroids, arranges rheumatology/medical follow-up

⇩ NO

⇩

Manage as mechanical/degenerative; give safety net for evolution of symptoms

Figure 13.3 Early inflammatory arthritis/spondyloarthritis/PMR-GCA (NICE 2024r and NICE 2024q).

PATIENT WITH REGIONAL MSK PAIN (SHOULDER/ELBOW/HIP/KNEE/FOOT)

⇩

History:
- Trauma vs non-trauma
- Occupation/sport/overuse
- Time course, aggravating movements
- Screen red flags (systemic, severe neuro, infection)

⇩

Significant trauma or red flags?

⇩ YES

⇩ Manage via trauma/urgent medical pathway

⇩ NO

⇩ Non-traumatic/overuse/degenerative

⇩

Non-traumatic and no red flags:
- Clinical diagnosis from pattern:
- Shoulder: RCRSP/frozen shoulder?
- Elbow: tennis/golfer's elbow?
- Hip: GTPS or OA?
- Knee: PF pain or OA?
- Foot/ankle: plantar fasciitis, Achilles tendinopathy?

⇩

FIRST-LINE MANAGEMENT:
- Reassurance and education
- Relative rest and load modification
- Condition-specific exercise (e.g. eccentric loading for Achilles; cuff loading for RCRSP)
- Simple analgesia as per NICE guidance

⇩

REVIEW AFTER 6–8 WEEKS

⇩ IMPROVING

⇩ Continue self-management; progress rehab

⇩ PERSISTENT/UNSURE

⇩ Consider imaging only if it will change management and/or referral to MSK/orthopaedics depending on local pathway

Figure 13.4 Soft tissue/MSK triage (upper or lower limb) (NICE NG226, 2022a; NICE NG193, 2020; GIRFT, 2023).

PATIENT WITH ACUTE TRAUMA TO LIMB OR SPINE

⇩

Primary survey: ABCDE if major trauma
Focused MSK assessment:
- Mechanism of injury
- Deformity, swelling, bruising
- Weight-bearing ability
- Neurovascular status

⇩

MAJOR TRAUMA?
(e.g. high-speed RTC, fall from height, multiple injuries, shock)

⇩ YES ⇩

Activate major trauma pathway/call 999

⇩ NO ⇩

For isolated limb/spine injury: apply decision rules:
- Ottawa ankle/knee rules etc.
- Consider X-ray when rules met or if high clinical suspicion

⇩

IMAGING and ACUTE MANAGEMENT:
- Immobilise suspected fractures
- Provide analgesia
- Refer to orthopaedics/fracture clinic

⇩

EARLY REHAB and FOLLOW-UP:
- Encourage safe early mobilisation where appropriate
- Arrange physiotherapy as needed
- Secondary prevention (falls, osteoporosis) in fragility fractures

Figure 13.5 Suspected fracture/trauma pathway (NICE NG37, NG38, NG40).

References

Abhishek, A., Roddy, E. and Doherty, M. (2017) 'Gout – a guide for the general and acute physicians', Clinical Medicine, 17(1), pp. 54–59.

Academy of Physical Medicine (2018) Clinical Model for Pattern Recognition in Pain Assessment. Available at: https://www.academyofphysicalmedicine.co.uk/wp-content/uploads/2018/10/26-Clinical-Model-for-Pattern-Recognition-in-Pain-Assessment.pdf (Accessed: 1st March 2025).

Albury, C. et al. (2022) 'Communication and behavioural approaches in musculoskeletal care', British Journal of General Practice, 72(718), pp. 240–242.

Aletaha, D. and Smolen, J.S. (2018) 'Diagnosis and management of rheumatoid arthritis: a review', Journal of the American Medical Association, 320(13), pp. 1360–1372.

Allen, A., Carville, S. and McKenna, F. (2018) 'Diagnosis and management of rheumatoid arthritis in adults: summary of updated NICE guidance', British Medical Journal, 362.

Almutairi, K. et al. (2021) 'The prevalence of rheumatoid arthritis: a systematic review of population-based studies', The Journal of Rheumatology, 48(5), pp. 669–676.

Alves, F. and Goncalo, M. (2019) 'Suspected inflammatory rheumatic diseases in patients presenting with skin rashes', Best Practice & Research Clinical Rheumatology, 33(4), p. 101440.

Ameer, M.A. et al. (2022) 'An overview of systemic lupus erythematosus (SLE) pathogenesis, classification, and management', Cureus, 14(10).

Ardern, C.L. et al. (2018) '2016 consensus statement on return to sport from the First World Congress in Sports Physical Therapy', British Journal of Sports Medicine, 52(8), pp. 506–517.

Aringer, M. et al. (2019) '2019 European League Against Rheumatism/American College of Rheumatology classification criteria for systemic lupus erythematosus', Arthritis & Rheumatology, 71(9), pp. 1400–1412.

Armstrong, A.D. et al. (2017) 'Management of elbow instability', Journal of the American Academy of Orthopaedic Surgeons, 25(9), pp. 647–657.

Asif, M.I. et al. (2023) 'Connective tissue disorders and eye: a review and recent updates', Indian Journal of Ophthalmology, 71(6), pp. 2385–2398.

Atroshi, I. et al. (2019) 'Treatment of carpal tunnel syndrome', The Lancet, 393(10174), pp. 1298–1307.

Bagnall, K.M., Harris, P.F. and Jones, P.R. (2008) 'A radiographic study of the human thoracic spine', Spine, 33(9), pp. 953–959.

Beaufils, P. et al. (2017) 'Surgical management of degenerative meniscus lesions: the 2016 ESSKA meniscus consensus', Knee Surgery, Sports Traumatology, Arthroscopy, 25(2), pp. 335–346.

Beitzel, K. et al. (2014) 'Biomechanics of the rotator cuff', Knee Surgery, Sports Traumatology, Arthroscopy, 22(2), pp. 226–236.

Bennett, M.I. et al. (2016) 'The S-LANSS score', Journal of Pain, 6(3), pp. 149–158.

Bentohami, A. et al. (2014) 'Incidence and characteristics of distal radial fractures in an urban population in The Netherlands', European Journal of Trauma and Emergency Surgery, 40(3), pp. 357–361.

Berwick, R., Barker, C., Goebel, A. and Guideline Development Group (2022) 'The diagnosis of fibromyalgia syndrome', Clinical Medicine, 22(6), pp. 570–574.

Bessen, T. et al. (2009) 'Implementation of the Ottawa ankle rules', British Medical Journal, 339, b3056.

Blackwell, J.R., Hay, B.A., Bolt, A.M. and Hay, S.M. (2014) 'Olecranon bursitis: a systematic overview', Shoulder & Elbow, 6(3), pp. 182–190.

Blyth F.M. et al. (2019) 'The global burden of musculoskeletal pain—where to from here?', American Journal of Public Health, 109(1), pp. 35–40.

BMJ Best Practice (2023) Dupuytren Contracture. Available at: https://bestpractice.bmj.com/topics/en-gb/983 (Accessed: 9th December 2025).

Bogduk, N. (2012) Clinical and Radiological Anatomy of the Lumbar Spine. 5th edn. Edinburgh: Churchill Livingstone/Elsevier

Bohn, R. et al. (2018) 'Incidence and prevalence of axial spondyloarthritis: methodologic challenges and gaps in the literature', Clinical and Experimental Rheumatology, 36(2), pp. 263–274.

Borghi, C. et al. (2020) 'Hyperuricaemia and gout in cardiovascular, metabolic and kidney disease', European Journal of Internal Medicine, 80, pp. 1–11.

Brady, O.J., Ginn, K.A., Murrell, G.A.C. and Bokor, D.J. (2020) 'Adhesive capsulitis: current diagnosis and management', Journal of Orthopaedic & Sports Physical Therapy, 50(7), pp. 380–398.

Briggs, A.M. et al. (2021) 'Consumers' experiences of back pain in primary care', Spine, 46(7), pp. E407–E417.

British Elbow and Shoulder Society (BESS) (2023) Patient care pathways and guidelines. Available at: https://bess.ac.uk/patient-care-pathways-and-guidelines/ (Accessed: 9th March 2025).

British Orthopaedic Association (BOA) (2022) Acute Compartment Syndrome. BOA Standards for Trauma (BOASt). Available at: https://www.boa.ac.uk (Accessed: 1st March 2025).

Bronfort, G. et al. (2016) 'Effectiveness of manual therapies: the UK evidence report', Chiropractic & Manual Therapies, 18(1), pp. 1–33.

Brooke-Wavell, K. et al. (2022) 'Strong, steady and straight: UK consensus statement on physical activity and exercise for osteoporosis', British Journal of Sports Medicine, 56(15), pp. 837–846.

Bullock, J. et al. (2018) 'Rheumatoid arthritis: a brief overview of the treatment', Journal of Medical Principles and Practice, 27(6), pp. 501–507.

Burahee, A.S. et al. (2021) 'Cubital tunnel syndrome', EFORT Open Reviews, 6(9), pp. 743–750.

Buttgereit, F. et al. (2024) 'Osteoporosis and fracture risk are multifactorial in patients with inflammatory rheumatic diseases', Nature Reviews Rheumatology, 20(7), pp. 417–431.

Cagnie, B. et al. (2013) 'Risk factors for neck pain among office workers', European Spine Journal, 22(5), pp. 1050–1057.

Carroll, L.J. et al. (2009) 'Course and prognostic factors for neck pain in whiplash-associated disorders', European Spine Journal, 17(Suppl 1), pp. 75–82.

Childs, J.D. et al. (2008) 'Neck pain: clinical practice guidelines linked to the ICF', Journal of Orthopaedic & Sports Physical Therapy, 38(9), pp. A1–A34.

Christie NHS Foundation Trust (2016) Briefing Paper: Use of Red Flags to Identify Serious Spinal Pathology. Available at: https://www.christie.nhs.uk/media/31nmrhdn/briefing-paper-use-of-red-flags-to-identify-serious-spinal-pathology-updated-jan-2016-1.pdf (Accessed: 9th December 2025).

Clarkson, H. (2020) Musculoskeletal Assessment: Joint Range of Motion, Muscle Testing, and Function. Philadelphia: Lippincott Williams & Wilkins.

Coombes, B.K., Bisset, L. and Vicenzino, B. (2015) 'Management of lateral elbow tendinopathy', The Lancet, 385(9987), pp. 1947–1956.

Cortet, B. et al. (2024) 'Similarities and differences between European guidelines for the management of postmenopausal osteoporosis', Archives of Osteoporosis, 19(1), p. 84.

Court, C., Mansour, E. and Bouthors, C. (2017) 'Thoracic disc herniation: surgical outcomes', Orthopaedics & Traumatology: Surgery & Research, 103(1), pp. S31–S37.

Court-Brown, C.M. et al. (2015) Rockwood and Green's Fractures in Adults. 8th edn. Philadelphia: Wolters Kluwer.

Croskerry, P. (2009) 'Clinical cognition and diagnostic error', Advances in Health Sciences Education, 14(S1), pp. 27–35.

Crossley, K.M. et al. (2016) '2016 patellofemoral pain consensus statement from the 4th International Patellofemoral Pain Research Retreat, Manchester. Part 1:

terminology, definitions, clinical examination, natural history, patellofemoral osteoarthritis and patient-reported outcome measures', British Journal of Sports Medicine, 50(14), pp. 839–843.

Cuff, A. (2020) Clinical Reasoning in Musculoskeletal Practice. Edinburgh: Elsevier.

Dejaco, C. et al. (2015) '2015 recommendations for the management of polymyalgia rheumatica: a European League Against Rheumatism/American College of Rheumatology collaborative initiative', Annals of the Rheumatic Diseases, 74(10), pp. 1799–1807.

Dias, J.J. et al. (2016) 'Dupuytren's contracture management', Journal of Hand Surgery (European Volume), 41(7), pp. 689–696.

Diercks, R. et al. (2014) 'Guideline for diagnosis and treatment of subacromial pain syndrome', Acta Orthopaedica, 85(3), pp. 314–322.

Dijkstra, H.P. et al. (2020) 'Return to play in elite sport: a systematic review', British Journal of Sports Medicine, 54(2), pp. 79–84.

Donskov, A.O. et al. (2023) 'An international survey of current management practices for polymyalgia rheumatica by general practitioners and rheumatologists', Rheumatology, 62(8), pp. 2797–2805.

Downie, A. et al. (2013) 'Red flags to screen for malignancy and fracture in patients with low back pain', British Medical Journal, 347, f7095.

Dubois, B. and Esculier, J.F. (2020) 'Soft-tissue injuries simply need PEACE and LOVE', British Journal of Sports Medicine, 54(2), pp. 72–73.

Edwards, R.R. et al. (2016) 'The role of psychosocial processes in the development and maintenance of chronic pain', The Journal of Pain, 17(9), pp. T70–T92.

Elshahawy, E. et al. (2022) 'Overlap of pain character in patients with inflammatory back pain versus chronic mechanical back pain', The Egyptian Journal of Hospital Medicine, 89(1), pp. 5375–5378.

Elstein, A.S., Shulman, L.S. and Sprafka, S.A. (1978) Medical Problem Solving: An analysis of clinical reasoning. Cambridge, MA: Harvard University Press.

Elwyn, G. et al. (2020) 'The three-talk model for shared decision making', British Medical Journal, 368, l6985.

Espígol-Frigolé, G. et al. (2023) 'Polymyalgia rheumatica', The Lancet, 402(10411), pp. 1459–1472.

Eva, K.W. (2005) 'Clinical reasoning: what every teacher needs to know', Medical Education, 39(1), pp. 98–106.

Falasinnu, T. et al. (2022) 'The problem of pain in rheumatology: clinical profiles associated with concomitant diagnoses with chronic overlapping pain conditions', ACR Open Rheumatology, 4(10), pp. 890–896.

Fanouriakis, A. et al. (2021) 'Update on the diagnosis and management of systemic lupus erythematosus', Annals of the Rheumatic Diseases, 80(1), pp. 14–25.

Ferrara, C.A. et al. (2023) 'Towards early diagnosis of mixed connective tissue disease: updated perspectives', ImmunoTargets and Therapy, 12, pp. 79–89.

Finucane, L.M. et al. (2020) 'International framework for red flags for potential serious spinal pathologies', Journal of Orthopaedic & Sports Physical Therapy, 50(7), pp. 350–372.

Foster, N.E. et al. (2018) 'Prevention and treatment of low back pain', The Lancet, 391(10137), pp. 2368–2383.

Freeman, G.K. et al. (2002) 'Evolving general practice consultation in Britain: issues of length and context', British Medical Journal, 324(7342), pp. 880–882.

Fuggle, N.R. et al. (2024) 'Evidence-based guideline for the management of osteoporosis in men', Nature Reviews Rheumatology, 20(4), pp. 241–251.

Gabel, C.P. et al. (2012) 'The Orebro Musculoskeletal Screening Questionnaire', Manual Therapy, 17(6), pp. 554–565.

GBD 2021 Low Back Pain Collaborators (2023) 'Global, regional, and national burden of low back pain, 1990–2020, its attributable risk factors, and projections to 2050: a systematic analysis of the Global Burden of Disease Study 2021', The Lancet Rheumatology, 5(6), pp. e316–e329.

Getting It Right First Time (GIRFT) (2020a) Community Musculoskeletal Services Handbook. London: NHS England.

Getting It Right First Time (GIRFT) (2023) Further Faster Community MSK Services Handbook. London: NHS England.

Gladman, D.D. et al. (2005) 'Psoriatic arthritis: epidemiology, clinical features, course, and outcome', Annals of the Rheumatic Diseases, 64(Suppl 2), pp. ii14–ii17.

Gossec, L. et al. (2020) 'EULAR recommendations for the management of psoriatic arthritis with pharmacological therapies: 2019 update', Annals of the Rheumatic Diseases, 79(6), pp. 700–712.

Goubran, A. and Tomlinson, J. (2023) 'Spinal infection: an overview', Journal of Trauma & Orthopaedics, 11(1), pp. 15–22.

Griffin, X.L. et al. (2016) 'Hip fracture management and outcomes', British Medical Journal, 354, i3515.

Gross, A. et al. (2016) 'Exercises for mechanical neck disorders', Cochrane Database of Systematic Reviews, (1), CD004250.

Gross, J., Fetto, J. and Rosen, E. (2015) Musculoskeletal Examination. Hoboken: John Wiley & Sons.

Hall, T., Robinson, K. and Fujinawa, O. (2010) 'Cervical flexion–rotation test reliability', Journal of Manipulative and Physiological Therapeutics, 33(7), pp. 513–517.

Hammam, N. et al. (2024) 'Clinical implications of seropositive and seronegative autoantibody status in rheumatoid arthritis patients: a comparative multicentre observational study', Rheumatology and Immunology Research, 5(1), pp. 57–65.

Hill, J.C. et al. (2022) 'Stratified care for musculoskeletal pain', The Lancet Rheumatology, 4(3), pp. e188–e197.

Hockings, R.L., McAuley, J.H. and Maher, C.G. (2008) 'Predictive ability of the Orebro Musculoskeletal Pain Questionnaire', Spine, 33(15), pp. E494–E500.

Hooper, T.L. et al. (2010) 'Thoracic outlet syndrome', Journal of Manual & Manipulative Therapy, 18(2), pp. 74–83.

Hui, M., Carr, A. and Cameron, S. (2017) 'British Society for Rheumatology and British Health Professionals in Rheumatology guideline for the management of gout', Rheumatology, 56(7), pp. 1056–1059.

Hunter, D.J. and Bierma-Zeinstra, S. (2022) 'Osteoarthritis', The Lancet, 393(10182), pp. 1745–1759.

Hysa, E. et al. (2025) 'Environmental factors in polymyalgia rheumatica and giant cell arteritis', Clinical and Experimental Rheumatology, 43, p. 100.

Illig, K.A. et al. (2016) Thoracic Outlet Syndrome. Softcover reprint of the 1st edn. London: Springer.

Ingram, T.A. et al. (2025) 'Delayed diagnosis of axial spondyloarthritis: the crucial role of primary care', British Journal of General Practice, 75(752), pp. 136–139.

Irving, G. et al. (2017) 'International variations in primary care physician consultation time: a systematic review of 67 countries', BMJ Open, 7(10), e017902.

Jay K, et al. (2018) 'Fear Avoidance Beliefs and Risk of Long-Term Sickness Absence: Prospective Cohort Study among Workers with Musculoskeletal Pain', Pain Research and Treatment, 8347120.

Jenkinson, T. et al. (1994) 'Defining spinal mobility in ankylosing spondylitis: the Bath AS Metrology Index', The Journal of Rheumatology, 21(9), pp. 1694–1698.

Jensen, R.K. et al. (2022) 'Clinical course of lumbar disc herniation', Spine Journal, 22(3), pp. 403–414.

Jones, E.A. et al. (2024) 'Management of fibromyalgia: an update', Biomedicines, 12(6), p. 1266.

Jones, M. et al. (2019) 'Thoracic outlet syndrome: comprehensive review', Pain Therapy, 8(1), pp. 5–18.

Josefsson, P.O. et al. (2018) 'Anterior shoulder dislocation management', Journal of Bone and Joint Surgery, 100(6), pp. 475–485.

Kalichman, L. et al. (2009) 'Spondylolysis and spondylolisthesis', Spine, 34(2), pp. 199–205.

Karran, E., McAuley, J.H. and Traeger, A.C. (2022) 'Red flags gone missing', Lancet Rheumatology, 4(5), pp. e341–e350.

Kay, J. and Upchurch, K.S. (2012) 'ACR/EULAR 2010 rheumatoid arthritis classification criteria', Rheumatology, 51(Suppl 6), pp. v5–v9.

Kearon, C. et al. (2019) 'Diagnosis and management of venous thromboembolism', Chest, 154(2), pp. 315–335.

Kurtz, S., Silverman, J. and Draper, J. (2017) Teaching and Learning Communication Skills in Medicine. 2nd edn. Oxford: Radcliffe.

Lamb, J. et al. (2012) 'One in a Million study: UK primary care consultations database', British Journal of General Practice, 62(605), pp. e345–e356.

Lewis, J.S. (2016) 'Rotator cuff related shoulder pain: assessment and management', British Journal of Sports Medicine, 50(5), pp. 298–300.

Lewis, J.S., McCreesh, K., Roy, J.S. and Ginn, K.A. (2015) 'Rotator cuff related shoulder pain', British Journal of Sports Medicine, 49(7), pp. 405–409.

Linton, S.J. and Shaw, W.S. (2011) 'Early identification and management of psychological risk factors in low back pain', Physical Therapy, 91(5), pp. 737–753.

Littlewood, C., May, S. and Walters, S. (2020) 'Clinical tests for rotator cuff pathology', Musculoskeletal Science and Practice, 50, 102262.

Longo, U.G. et al. (2011) 'Management of rotator cuff tears', British Medical Bulletin, 99(1), pp. 63–87.

Luime, J. et al. (2004) 'Prevalence and incidence of shoulder pain in the general population: a systematic review', Scandinavian Journal of Rheumatology, 33(2), pp. 73–81.

Macfarlane, G.J. et al. (2017) 'EULAR revised recommendations for the management of fibromyalgia', Annals of the Rheumatic Diseases, 76(2), pp. 318–328.

Macleod, J. (2018) Macleod's Clinical Examination. 14th edn. Edinburgh: Elsevier.

Magee, D.J. (2021) Orthopedic Physical Assessment. 7th edn. St. Louis, MO: Elsevier.

Mahadevan, D. et al. (2015) 'Diagnostic accuracy of clinical tests for Morton's neuroma compared with ultrasonography', Journal of Foot and Ankle Surgery, 54(4), pp. 549–553.

Maini, M. et al. (2020) 'A global perspective on the challenges and opportunities in learning about rheumatic and musculoskeletal diseases in undergraduate medical education', Clinical Rheumatology, 39, pp. 627–642.

Makkouk, A.H. et al. (2008) 'Carpal tunnel syndrome: a review', Orthopedic Clinics of North America, 39(2), pp. 173–184.

Mathews, C.J. et al. (2008) 'Management of septic arthritis: a systematic review', Postgraduate Medical Journal, 84(991), pp. 265–270.

Mathews, J.A. et al. (2021) 'Early inflammatory arthritis recognition', British Journal of General Practice, 71(702), pp. 34–36.

McCormick, J. et al. (2020) 'Cervical spondylotic myelopathy: diagnosis and management', Journal of the American Board of Family Medicine, 33(2), pp. 303–313.

McSweeney, S.C. and Cichero, M. (2015) 'Tarsal tunnel syndrome — a narrative literature review', Foot, 25(4), pp. 244–250.

Medicines and Healthcare Products Regulatory Agency (MHRA) (2019) Fluoroquinolone Antibiotics: Updated Advice on Risk of Disabling and Potentially Long-Lasting or Irreversible Side Effects. Drug Safety Update. London: MHRA.

Meinke, A. et al. (2025) 'Fear avoidance beliefs are associated with reduction of back movements', Pain Reports, 10(3), e1290.

Mellor, R. et al. (2018) 'Education plus exercise versus corticosteroid injection use versus a wait and see approach on global outcome and pain from gluteal tendinopathy', British Medical Journal, 361, k1662.

Milewski, M.D. et al. (2019) 'Anterior cruciate ligament injuries in young athletes', Journal of the American Academy of Orthopaedic Surgeons, 27(6), pp. 194–202.

Mitchell, C. et al. (2005) 'Shoulder pain: diagnosis and management in primary care', British Medical Journal, 331, pp. 1124–1128.

Mont, M.A. et al. (2015) 'Osteonecrosis of the femoral head', The Journal of Bone and Joint Surgery, 97(23), pp. 1928–1939.

Musculoskeletal Association of Chartered Physiotherapists (MACP) (2016) Cauda Equina Syndrome Information Card. Available at: https://www.macpweb.org/learning-resources/cauda-equina-information-cards.aspx (Accessed: 1st March 2025).

National Institute for Health and Care Excellence (NICE) (2015) Suspected Cancer: Recognition and Referral [NG12]. Available at: https://www.nice.org.uk/guidance/ng12 (Accessed: 1st March 2025).

National Institute for Health and Care Excellence (NICE) (2016a) Low Back Pain and Sciatica in Over 16s: Assessment and Management [NG59]. Available at: https://www.nice.org.uk/guidance/ng59 (Accessed: 1st March 2025).

National Institute for Health and Care Excellence (NICE) (2016b) Fractures (Non-Complex): Assessment and Management [NG38]. Available at: https://www.nice.org.uk/guidance/ng38 (Accessed: 1st March 2025).

National Institute for Health and Care Excellence (NICE) (2016c) Fractures (Complex): Assessment and Management [NG37]. Available at: https://www.nice.org.uk/guidance/ng37 (Accessed: 1st March 2025).

National Institute for Health and Care Excellence (NICE) (2016d) Major Trauma: Assessment and Management [NG40]. Available at: https://www.nice.org.uk/guidance/ng40 (Accessed: 1st March 2025).

National Institute for Health and Care Excellence (NICE) (2017) Spondyloarthritis in Over 16s: Diagnosis and Management [NG65]. Available at: https://www.nice.org.uk/guidance/ng65 (Accessed: 1st March 2025).

National Institute for Health and Care Excellence (NICE) (2018) Rheumatoid Arthritis in Adults: Management [NG100]. Available at: https://www.nice.org.uk/guidance/ng100 (Accessed: 1st March 2025).

National Institute for Health and Care Excellence (NICE) (2020) Chronic Pain (Primary and Secondary) in Over 16s: Assessment and Management of Chronic Primary Pain [NG193]. Available at: https://www.nice.org.uk/guidance/ng193 (Accessed: 1st March 2025).

National Institute for Health and Care Excellence (NICE) (2021a) Shared Decision Making [NG197]. Available at: https://www.nice.org.uk/guidance/ng197 (Accessed: 1st March 2025).

National Institute for Health and Care Excellence (NICE) (2021b) Suspected Neurological Conditions: Recognition and Referral [NG127]. Available at: https://www.nice.org.uk/guidance/ng127 (Accessed: 1st March 2025).

National Institute for Health and Care Excellence (NICE) (2022a) Osteoarthritis in Over 45s: Diagnosis and Management [NG226]. Available at: https://www.nice.org.uk/guidance/ng226 (Accessed: 1st March 2025).

National Institute for Health and Care Excellence (NICE) (2022b) Gout: Diagnosis and Management [NG219]. Available at: https://www.nice.org.uk/guidance/ng219 (Accessed: 1st March 2025).

National Institute for Health and Care Excellence (NICE) (2023a) Metastatic Spinal Cord Compression in Adults: Risk Assessment, Diagnosis and Management [NG234]. Available at: https://www.nice.org.uk/guidance/ng234 (Accessed: 1st March 2025).

National Institute for Health and Care Excellence (NICE) (2023b) Venous Thromboembolic Diseases: Diagnosis, Management and Thrombophilia Testing [NG158]. Available at: https://www.nice.org.uk/guidance/ng158 (Accessed: 1st March 2025).

National Institute for Health and Care Excellence (NICE) (2023c) Neck Pain – Non-Specific. Clinical Knowledge Summary. Available at: https://cks.nice.org.uk/topics/neck-pain-non-specific/ (Accessed: 1st March 2025).

National Institute for Health and Care Excellence (NICE) (2024) Musculoskeletal Conditions. Available at: https://www.nice.org.uk/guidance/conditions-and-diseases/musculoskeletal-conditions (Accessed: 1st March 2025).

National Institute for Health and Care Excellence (NICE) (2024a) Musculoskeletal – Overview. Clinical Knowledge Summary. Available at: https://cks.nice.org.uk/topics/musculoskeletal (Accessed: 1st March 2025).

National Institute for Health and Care Excellence (NICE) (2024b) Shoulder Pain. Clinical Knowledge Summary. Available at: https://cks.nice.org.uk/topics/shoulder-pain (Accessed: 1st March 2025).

National Institute for Health and Care Excellence (NICE) (2024c) Neck Pain – Cervical Radiculopathy. Clinical Knowledge Summary. Available at: https://cks.nice.org.uk/topics/neck-pain-cervical-radiculopathy (Accessed: 1st March 2025).

National Institute for Health and Care Excellence (NICE) (2024d) Back Pain – Low (without Radiculopathy). Clinical Knowledge Summary. Available at: https://cks.nice.org.uk/topics/back-pain-low-without-radiculopathy (Accessed: 1st March 2025).

National Institute for Health and Care Excellence (NICE) (2024e) Knee Pain – Assessment. Clinical Knowledge Summary. Available at: https://cks.nice.org.uk/topics/knee-pain-assessment (Accessed: 1st March 2025).

National Institute for Health and Care Excellence (NICE) (2024f) Hip Pain – Assessment. Clinical Knowledge Summary. Available at: https://cks.nice.org.uk/topics/hip-pain-assessment (Accessed: 1st March 2025).

National Institute for Health and Care Excellence (NICE) (2024g) Greater Trochanteric Pain Syndrome. Clinical Knowledge Summary. Available at: https://cks.nice.org.uk/topics/greater-trochanteric-pain-syndrome (Accessed: 1st March 2025).

National Institute for Health and Care Excellence (NICE) (2024h) Achilles Tendinopathy. Clinical Knowledge Summary. Available at: https://cks.nice.org.uk/topics/achilles-tendinopathy (Accessed: 1st March 2025).

National Institute for Health and Care Excellence (NICE) (2024i) Plantar Fasciitis. Clinical Knowledge Summary. Available at: https://cks.nice.org.uk/topics/plantar-fasciitis (Accessed: 1st March 2025).

National Institute for Health and Care Excellence (NICE) (2024j) Carpal Tunnel Syndrome. Clinical Knowledge Summary. Available at: https://cks.nice.org.uk/topics/carpal-tunnel-syndrome (Accessed: 1st March 2025).

National Institute for Health and Care Excellence (NICE) (2024k) Tennis Elbow. Clinical Knowledge Summary. Available at: https://cks.nice.org.uk/topics/tennis-elbow (Accessed: 1st March 2025).

National Institute for Health and Care Excellence (NICE) (2024l) De Quervain's Tenosynovitis. Clinical Knowledge Summary. Available at: https://cks.nice.org.uk/topics/de-quervains-tenosynovitis (Accessed: 1st March 2025).

National Institute for Health and Care Excellence (NICE) (2024m) Trigger Finger. Clinical Knowledge Summary. Available at: https://cks.nice.org.uk/topics/trigger-finger (Accessed: 1st March 2025).

National Institute for Health and Care Excellence (NICE) (2024o) Osteoporosis – Prevention of Fragility Fractures. Clinical Knowledge Summary. Available at: https://cks.nice.org.uk/topics/osteoporosis-prevention-of-fragility-fractures (Accessed: 1st March 2025).

National Institute for Health and Care Excellence (NICE) (2024p) Myalgia. Clinical Knowledge Summary. Available at: https://cks.nice.org.uk/topics/myalgia (Accessed: 1st March 2025).

National Institute for Health and Care Excellence (NICE) (2024q) Polymyalgia Rheumatica. Clinical Knowledge Summary. Available at: https://cks.nice.org.uk/topics/polymyalgia-rheumatica (Accessed: 1st March 2025).

National Institute for Health and Care Excellence (NICE) (2024r) Giant Cell Arteritis. Clinical Knowledge Summary. Available at: https://cks.nice.org.uk/topics/giant-cell-arteritis (Accessed: 1st March 2025).

National Institute for Health and Care Excellence (NICE) (2024s) Falls – Risk Assessment. Clinical Knowledge Summary. Available at: https://cks.nice.org.uk/topics/falls-risk-assessment (Accessed: 1st March 2025).

National Institute for Health and Care Excellence (NICE) (2025) Osteoarthritis: Management. Clinical Knowledge Summary. Available at: https://cks.nice.org.uk/topics/osteoarthritis (Accessed: 1st March 2025).

Nepple, J.J. et al. (2018) 'Femoroacetabular impingement', Journal of the American Academy of Orthopaedic Surgeons, 26(12), pp. 414–424.

Ng, I. and Chan, K. (2024) 'Physicians, know thy patient: a study on patient-centred medical care', International Journal of Medical Research, 32(1).

NHS Digital (2022) Back Pain Prevalence in Adults. Leeds: NHS Digital.

NHS England (2021) Musculoskeletal Health: Economic and Service Impact. London: NHS England.

Nicholas, M.K. et al. (2011) 'Psychological risk factors and early management', Pain, 152(5), pp. 1145–1149.

Niemantsverdriet, E. and Van der Helm-van Mil, A.H.M. (2018) 'Imaging detected tenosynovitis of metacarpophalangeal and wrist joints: an increasingly recognised characteristic of rheumatoid arthritis', Clinical and Experimental Rheumatology, 36(Suppl 114), pp. 131–138.

Norman, G. (2005) 'Research in clinical reasoning: past history and current trends', Medical Education, 39(4), pp. 418–427.

Nouri, A. et al. (2015) 'Degenerative cervical myelopathy: epidemiology, genetics and pathogenesis', Spine, 40(12), pp. E675–E693.

Office for National Statistics (ONS) (2023) Sickness Absence in the UK Labour Market: 2023. Available at: https://www.ons.gov.uk/employmentandlabourmarket/peopleinwork/labourproductivity/articles/sicknessabsenceinthelabourmarket/2023 (Accessed: 1st March 2025).

Oliveira, C.B. et al. (2021) 'Clinical practice guidelines for the management of non-specific musculoskeletal pain', Pain, 162(7), pp. 1966–1975.

Papalia, R. et al. (2020) 'Meniscal injuries: treatment and outcomes', Knee Surgery, Sports Traumatology, Arthroscopy, 28(2), pp. 370–380.

Personalised Care Institute (2020b) Dupuytren's Contracture: Decision Support Tool. Available at: https://www.personalisedcareinstitute.org.uk (Accessed: 9th December 2025).

Petty, N.J. (2011) Musculoskeletal Examination and Assessment: A Handbook for Therapists. 4th edn. Edinburgh: Elsevier Churchill Livingstone.

Pincus, T. et al. (2002) 'Psychological predictors of chronicity/disability in low back pain', Spine, 27(5), pp. E109–E120.

Poddubnyy, D. et al. (2021) 'Axial involvement in psoriatic arthritis: an update for rheumatologists', Seminars in Arthritis and Rheumatism, 51(4), pp. 880–887.

Public Health England and Health Education England (2016) Making Every Contact Count (MECC): Consensus Statement. Leeds: Public Health England. Available at: https://assets.publishing.service.gov.uk/government/uploads/system/uploads/

attachment_data/file/769486/Making_Every_Contact_Count_Consensus_Statement.pdf (Accessed: 1st March 2025).
Ramiro, S. et al. (2023) 'ASAS-EULAR recommendations for the management of axial spondyloarthritis', Annals of the Rheumatic Diseases, 82(1), pp. 19–34.
Ramon, A. et al. (2022) 'Predictive factors of giant cell arteritis in polymyalgia rheumatica patients', Journal of Clinical Medicine, 11(24), p. 7412.
Rasenberg, N. et al. (2018) 'Foot orthoses for plantar heel pain', British Journal of Sports Medicine, 52(5), pp. 322–328.
Roddy, E., Jordan, K.M. and Giles, I. (2024) 'Diagnosis and management of gout: are the British Society for Rheumatology and National Institute for Health and Care Excellence guidelines both needed?', Rheumatology Advances in Practice, 8(1).
Rosenberg, N. et al. (2020) 'Hand fracture management', Journal of Hand Surgery, 45(4), pp. 345–352.
Royal Osteoporosis Society (2022) Guidance on Managing Symptoms of Vertebral Fractures. Bath: Royal Osteoporosis Society.
Salaffi, F. et al. (2021) 'Rheumatoid arthritis disease activity assessment in routine care: performance of the most widely used composite disease activity indices and patient-reported outcome measures', Acta Bio Medica, 92(4), pp. 202–238.
Salisbury, C. et al. (2022a) 'Measuring the complexity of general practice consultations', British Journal of General Practice, 72(605), pp. e423–e430.
Salisbury, C. et al. (2022b) 'Primary care management of musculoskeletal pain', British Medical Journal, 338, b1449.
Salmon, P. and Young, B. (2011) Clinical Communication Skills. Oxford: Oxford University Press.
Schini, M. et al. (2024) 'An overview of the use of the fracture risk assessment tool (FRAX) in osteoporosis', Journal of Endocrinological Investigation, 47(3), pp. 501–511.
Schroeder, J.D. and Varacallo, M.A. (2024) Smith fracture. StatPearls. Available at: https://www.ncbi.nlm.nih.gov/books/NBK547714/ (Accessed: March 2025).
Siddiqui, S. et al. (2020) 'Cauda equina compression in metastatic prostate cancer', BMJ Case Reports 17.
Siddle, H.J. et al. (2023) 'Opportunities and challenges in early diagnosis of rheumatoid arthritis in general practice', British Journal of General Practice, 73(729), pp. 152–154.
Siegel, C.H. and Sammaritano, L.R. (2024) 'Systemic lupus erythematosus: a review', Journal of the American Medical Association, 331(17), pp. 1480–1491.
Silbernagel, K.G., Hanlon, S. and Sprague, A. (2020) 'Current clinical concepts: conservative management of Achilles tendinopathy', Journal of Athletic Training, 55(5), pp. 438–447.
Silverman, J., Kurtz, S. and Draper, J. (2013) Skills for Communicating with Patients. 3rd edn. London: Radcliffe Publishing.

Singh, J.A. et al. (2020) 'ACR guideline for management of gout', Arthritis Care & Research, 72(6), pp. 744–760.

Srinivasan, S. et al. (2019) 'The problematic nature of fibromyalgia diagnosis in the community', ACR Open Rheumatology, 1(1), pp. 43–51.

Standring, S. (2021) Gray's Anatomy: The Anatomical Basis of Clinical Practice. 42nd edn. London: Elsevier.

Stearns, Z.R. et al. (2021) 'Screening for yellow flags in orthopaedic physical therapy', Journal of Orthopaedic & Sports Physical Therapy, 51(9), pp. 459–469.

Stewart, M.A. (2005) 'Effective physician–patient communication and health outcomes', Patient Education and Counselling, 52(3), pp. 123–132.

Stone, M.A. et al. (2009) 'Significance of clinical evaluation of the metacarpophalangeal joint in relation to synovial/bone pathology in rheumatoid and psoriatic arthritis detected by magnetic resonance imaging', The Journal of Rheumatology, 36(12), pp. 2751–2757.

Swadling, W. et al. (2024) 'Cauda equina syndrome', Surgery (Oxford), 42(6), pp. 424–430.

Szekanecz, Z. et al. (2021) 'Autoinflammation and autoimmunity across rheumatic and musculoskeletal diseases', Nature Reviews Rheumatology, 17(10), pp. 585–595.

Talley, N.J. and O'Connor, S. (2021) Clinical Examination: A Systematic Guide to Physical Diagnosis. 8th edn. Chatswood: Elsevier.

Teissier, V. et al. (2019) 'Importance of early diagnosis and care in knee dislocations associated with vascular injuries', Annals of Vascular Surgery, 61, pp. 238–245.

Theodorou, A., Komnos, G. and Hantes, M. (2023) 'Patellar tendinopathy', Archives of Orthopaedic and Trauma Surgery, 143(11), pp. 6695–6705.

Thomas, L.C. et al. (2019) 'Risk factors for cervical arterial dysfunction', Manual Therapy, 24, pp. 11–19.

Tillett, W. et al. (2021) 'Treatment of psoriatic arthritis with biologic and targeted synthetic DMARDs: British Society for Rheumatology guideline scope', Rheumatology, 60(4), pp. 1588–1592.

Turnpenney, J. et al. (2015) 'Developing an early alert system for metastatic spinal cord compression (MSCC): red flag credit cards', Primary Health Care Research & Development, 16(1), pp. 14–20.

Vambe, S.D. et al. (2024) 'Crystals of pain: navigating gout and its management', SA Pharmaceutical Journal, 91(4), pp. 26–32.

Van der Heijde, D. et al. (2017) '2016 update of the ASAS-EULAR management recommendations for axial spondyloarthritis', Annals of the Rheumatic Diseases, 76(6), pp. 978–991.

Van der Windt, D.A.W.M. et al. (2010) 'Shoulder disorders in general practice', British Medical Journal, 341, c5659.

Versus Arthritis (2023) The State of Musculoskeletal Health 2023: Arthritis and Other Musculoskeletal Conditions in Numbers. Chesterfield: Versus Arthritis. Available at: https://www.versusarthritis.org/media/duybjusg/versus-arthritis-state-msk-musculoskeletal-health-2023pdf.pdf (Accessed: 1st March 2025).

Vilgran, M., Patel, R. and Chan, D. (2023) 'Neurological screening in primary care', Journal of Primary Care & Community Health, 14, p. 21501319231122345.

Vlaeyen, J.W.S. and Linton, S.J. (2000) 'Fear-avoidance and chronic musculoskeletal pain', Pain, 85(3), pp. 317–332.

Vleeming, A. et al. (2012) 'The sacroiliac joint: an overview of its anatomy, function and potential clinical implications', Journal of Anatomy, 221(6), pp. 537–567.

Waddell, G. et al. (1993) 'Fear Avoidance Beliefs Questionnaire (FABQ)', Pain, 52(2), pp. 157–168.

Wang, J.H.C. et al. (2017) 'Tendon mechanobiology', Journal of Orthopaedic Research, 35(3), pp. 518–528.

Weaver, J.S. et al. (2021) 'Gouty arthropathy: review of clinical manifestations and treatment, with emphasis on imaging', Journal of Clinical Medicine, 11(1), p. 166.

Willers, C. et al. and SCOPE Review Panel (2022) 'Osteoporosis in Europe: a compendium of country-specific reports', Archives of Osteoporosis, 17(1), p. 23.

Willy, R. W. et al. (2019) 'Patellofemoral pain: clinical practice guidelines linked to the International Classification of Functioning, Disability and Health from the Academy of Orthopaedic Physical Therapy of the American Physical Therapy Association', Journal of Orthopaedic & Sports Physical Therapy, 49(9), pp. CPG1–CPG95.

Wilson, A. and Childs, S. (2002) 'Consultation length and outcomes in general practice', British Journal of General Practice, 52, pp. 1012–1020.

Wolf, J.M., Sturdivant, R.X. and Owens, B.D. (2009) 'Incidence of de Quervain's tenosynovitis in a young, active population', Journal of Hand Surgery, 34(1), pp. 112–115.

World Health Organization (WHO) (1986) Cancer Pain Relief. Geneva: World Health Organization. Available at: https://apps.who.int/iris/bitstream/handle/10665/43944/9241561009_eng.pdf (Accessed: 1st March 2025).

Yazigi Junior, J.A. et al. (2021) 'Supraspinatus tears: predictability of magnetic resonance imaging findings based on clinical examination', Journal of Shoulder and Elbow Surgery, 30(8), pp. 1834–1843.

Zabotti, A. et al. (2020) 'From psoriasis to psoriatic arthritis: insights from imaging on the transition to psoriatic arthritis and implications for arthritis prevention', Current Rheumatology Reports, 22, pp. 1–9.

Zhang, W. et al. (2009) 'EULAR evidence-based recommendations for the diagnosis of hand osteoarthritis: report of a task force of ESCISIT', Annals of the Rheumatic Diseases, 68(1), pp. 8–17.

Zusman, N.L. et al. (2022) 'Physical examination is predictive of cauda equina syndrome: MRI to rule out diagnosis is unnecessary', Global Spine Journal, 12(2), pp. 209–214.

Index

I

K

L

M

N

O

P

R

S

T